No Pause at All

Books by Louis Parrish, M.D.

No Pause at All
Cooking as Therapy

No Pause at All

Louis Parrish, M.D.

READER'S DIGEST PRESS
Distributed by Thomas Y. Crowell Company
New York, 1976

Library of Congress Cataloging in Publication Data

Parrish, Louis.
  No pause at all.

  Includes index.
  1. Climacteric. I. Title.
RC884.P37   618.1'72   75–31811
ISBN 0–88349–085–4

1   2   3   4   5   6   7   8   9   10

To William D. Wheat, M.D.

Acknowledgments

The author wishes to express his thanks to Phyllis Schindler and George Kuharsky for their help in the preparation of this manuscript; to John Jewell, M.D. for sharing his extensive knowledge; and to Nancy Kelly, an understanding editor and friend.

Contents

Introduction

"Middle age" is often approached with distaste. Contemporary men and women reflect the increasingly fashionable notion that all the "middles" of life—middle class, middle-of-the-road, midway, even middle America—must be rejected. Middle is thought to be another word for nowhere at all—nothing.

It could be argued that this last view is correct. Middle *is* nothing—except in relation to something else. Without youth on the one hand and old age on the other, middle age could not exist. This sandwiched position is in large measure responsible for the "crisis" nature of middle age—a regret for the lost optimism and adventure of youth and a pessimism and fear of old age ahead. The attitude of modern society has not helped this situation.

With the breakdown of the family structure, the elderly have been affected even more than the young. The extended family, where Grandma played an important role in rearing children, has disappeared. Now Grandma is more likely to be tucked away in what we euphemistically call a "home." And Grandpa, who once dropped dead on the job, is pushed aside with a pat on the back and a gold watch at age sixty-five, or even younger. No wonder, then, the the middle years are often over-shadowed by a morbid fear not so much of dying as of living—but living *old*; and living empty.

Rays of hope are creeping through this gloomy picture, however. Though today more and more younger people are in important positions of policy making, they are mature enough to realize what is happening to their elders—whom they will someday replace. Though their concern may be selfish, it is beneficial for the elderly. We depend on such social and political forces, as well as scientific forces, to correct the distortions that appear from time to time. Take, for example, the declining birthrate. The median age of Americans will continue to rise, and what is now a misunderstood, confused minority group will soon be not a minority at all. Middle age, as a way of life as well as a time of life, will be recognized, even prized, for the productive period it can and should be.

Certainly a preoccupation with youth is not new to our society. From Greek statuary to Shakespeare's sonnets, to more modern works, the idealization of youth is a part of our aesthetic heritage. What has changed is our attitude toward the virtues of age. An appreciation, even veneration, of age and its primary value—the wisdom of experience—was once a prerequisite for civilization, even for life itself. Tribal man could ill afford the loss of wisdom and experience in the daily struggle for food and shelter. Even today, primitive societies retain a productive position for their old. It is only our modern "civilization" that has relegated the aged to its back rooms.

This is a foolish attitude that cannot be tolerated. Fortunately, both general and scientific forces are at work to make middle age a fulfilling and gracious transition to a rewarding old age. Preventive medicine is one of these. There is increasing research in controlling and counteracting the problems of middle age. In women especially, a great measure of the physical *and* psychological discomforts of middle age are produced by nothing more complicated than a deficiency of the hormone estrogen. The attitude of both patients and physicians toward the use of this hormone and its potential benefits is being reappraised, and today thousands of women are discovering the revitalizing properties of estrogen replacement therapy, ERT.

For men as well, there have been significant breakthroughs in the problems of middle age. Not only has medical science begun to identify and quantify these problems, but—best of all—has steadily been coming up with answers.

Most of this has occurred in such a short span of time as to be practically encompassed by the lifetime of those now in their middle years. The primary medical discoveries have come so fast that in many ways the weakest link in the chain of medical care has been the dissemination of information—from scientist to physician and from physician to patient. That is the purpose of this volume: to present the information in applicable form, then *use* it—in the fullest sense of the word.

My own professional career has spanned more than two decades, and during that time I have become increasingly involved in the diseases and disorders of middle age. My interest was first sparked many years ago, when I was a resident at a large Manhattan hospital and performed my first emergency autopsy. Lifting aside the sheet, I found the body of a pitifully wasted woman. She appeared to be in her late fifties, but according to the chart she was only forty-five. I know now (and there are few more poignant phrases in the English language than those three words) that this patient was a victim of severe hormone deficiency. Following a series of "female problems" and resultant complications, a radical hysterectomy had been performed, removing her uterus and ovaries. The lack of a uterus ended her fertility. But the removal of her ovaries, and the extreme hormone deficiency it produced, ended her life. With a little research, I understood that my autopsy patient was not the only victim of this deficiency. All women, if they live long enough, suffer a form of castration. By age fifty-five, the ovaries have almost inevitably reduced, or virtually ceased, their hormone secretions. Some research into female hormone replacement was being done at the time, and I decided that this was an area of medicine in which I wanted to get involved. After a tour of duty with the navy, I took a job with a large pharmaceutical house engaged in hormone replacement research. Later I joined the visiting staff of a New York hospital, under the tutelage of one of the giants of endrocrinology, Dr. Max Goldzieher. And soon, at his urging, I found myself with a part-time private practice.

One of my first patients was a Mrs. Peabody,* who came into my office displaying all the symptoms of an acute menopausal crisis. It took no genius to diagnose her conglomeration of hot flushes, sudden sweats, and general irritability—the popularly known effects of "the change." But it was genius—not my genius, of course, but that of tireless researchers—to offer her a "cure": a replacement for the hormone her ovaries could no longer manufacture. To Mrs. Peabody, it was indeed a "miracle."

---

*Throughout this book the names have been changed, but the substance of the case histories has been taken directly from my files.

Her friends thought so, too. Soon my part-time practice became full time, and full of middle-aged men and women. But it didn't take me long to discover my physician's feet of clay. Dealing with the medical problem was not always enough. I was struck with the realization that people need to have a doctor see them as a person as well as a disease. Without psychological assistance, no purely physical "cure" is sufficient. So I spent the next three years in a psychiatric residency.

For the last ten years, then, I've been dealing on a day-to-day basis with the inevitable changes, physical *and* psychological, that accompany middle life. And I've been able to tell each of my patients what I can tell each of my readers—it can actually be a change for the better.

But before we talk about the quality of the change, it's best to spend some time talking about what exactly is involved. This brings us to terminology, a new vocabulary for middle age.

Both men and women are subject, at some point in mid-life, to a variety of changes—physical, psychological, and social. To denote these changes and their symptoms, I use the term *climacteric*.

In the female, the climacteric is easily recognized by its common symptom, the natural cessation of the menses, the menopause. Surrounding the menopause may come the classic symptoms of "the change": physical symptoms like hot flushes and sweats as well as emotional difficulties—headaches, fatigue, insomnia. But whether these attendant troubles accompany the menopause or not, the climacteric has begun. And long after temporary symptoms associated with the menopause have passed, further climacteric complications are possible, subtle changes that may not produce symptoms for a decade or more.

The outlines of the male climacteric are more shadowy

than those of the female, since there is no common symptom, such as the menopause, to mark the transition. Still, definite physical and psychological transitions are taking place through the middle years in the male as well, and I hope as this volume progresses to bring them into proper perspective.

This, however, involves another kind of change: a change in attitude. To read this book indicates that you have already suspected that something can be done to prevent, control, and correct the potential disorders of middle age—and you're right. In this case forewarned is forearmed. Life *can* begin at forty or fifty or beyond—a different life, perhaps, but a new and vigorous one. It is my firm belief that youth—or the soundness of mind and body that youth symbolizes—need not be limited to the young. With knowledge and a little care, life can be lived to the fullest right through the middle years. There need be no pause at all—in your physical health, your sense of well-being, and your general involvement with life.

A New Life

Estrogen and Biological Change

For all of society's focus on aging and its effects, we seem to care little for the true facts on the subject. We give scant notice to the complexities of our physical existence as human beings; instead we are likely to compare ourselves to simpler life-forms. We see a mirror of ourselves in, say, a plant: from a tiny seedling grows the stem and leaves; the mature plant sends forth a bud which flowers, then fades; its reproductive purpose served, the plant dies.

This may be an apt metaphor with which to teach a child in kindergarten the facts of what we call the "life cycle." But to apply the same metaphor to human life is absurd.

The decline of the reproductive cycle is by no means the end of the human life cycle. Human beings continue to grow until the day they die. Of course there are changes—what would life be without them? But change can be, and should be, positive. Take a simple matter like the body's demand for food. The fact is that by middle age, the body usually requires less food to keep it going.

Some people find this distressing; it means they cannot indulge themselves at the same rate as previously and not expect to become overweight. But in light of our worldwide food shortage, we should be delighted, as a species, that adults need not consume the same quantities as adolescents to fuel their bodies.

The decline of physical strength is often deplored, yet it, too, is an appropriate change. Women who have gone through the hard physical labor of raising a family don't need—and shouldn't need—the same amount of strength in later years. Human beings who have made the technological strides we've seen in the last century *deserve* the leisure they have won. And with the decline of manual labor in favor of white-collar employment, people can continue productive careers decades longer than they might have even a century ago.

I'm not trying to suggest that there are no ill effects of aging; there are, some of them serious, all of them important. Arteries lose elasticity, glandular secretion is less synchronized, and nervous tissue becomes less responsive and sensitive. But such changes should not be considered abnormal.

These cells are not diseased. The fact is, they simply do not need to be as responsive as they once were. Growing old, like growing up, is a matter of biological development. Every cell and every organ is affected in some way, but this need not produce a symptom or pain, or even cause a temporary dysfunction. The general effect of age on the body and brain (and, indirectly, on the mind) varies from person to person, according to events in their life, their life-style, and their heredity. There are, of course, certain aspects of aging that are inevitable. Some apply primarily to men, some only to women, and some to both sexes. First let us discuss a change that is unique to women—the loss or deficiency of the female hormone estrogen.

Woman is the only animal with a menstrual cycle who is not capable of reproducing up until the time she dies. The human child, unlike the offspring of other animals, requires many years of care before it can be on its own. So by the laws of natural selection, the species of *Homo sapiens* whose female stopped reproducing at a point in life when she still had time to nurture her child to maturity was the species that survived. So the menopause evolved as a natural event.

Since pregnancy and delivery are more likely to be dangerous in a woman's later life, ovulation becomes a liability and the atrophy of the ovaries a practical solution to the problem. But along with this natural atrophy comes a decrease in the secretion of estrogen, which is vital to important biological functions. This estrogen deficiency can accelerate certain aspects of the aging process, but fortunately such a deficiency is not inevitable. Some women's ovaries do continue to furnish an adequate estrogen supply. But for the many women whose ovaries cease to supply enough, modern science has now found a solution.

To understand the full meaning of the atrophy of the ovaries we should consider their previous effect on a woman's life. The ovaries are formed from a group of cells, the germinal epithelium, that are segregated soon after conception. As the fetus develops they take their place in the pelvic cavity where they remain inconspicuous in size and activity until puberty, when they burst into action and turn a girl into a woman.

This magic is effected by a series of biological events that originate in the base of the brain, which is the center of our primitive animal nature. A message is sent to the master endocrine gland, the pituitary, to secrete hormones which specifically stimulate the ovaries. They respond by manufacturing their own hormone, which is carried by the bloodstream throughout the body. This hormone, estrogen, stimulates the growth of the breasts, womb, and vagina. In addition, the estrogen activates the hair follicles under the arm and around the pubis, while increasing the deposition of fat around the hips and in the breasts.

As a young girl's body fills out, the first of the eggs in her ovaries reaches maturity. As it matures, the follicle housing the egg secretes estrogen to such a level that it slows the pituitary's production of the stimulating hormone. The estrogen thickens the lining of the womb (the endometrium), preparing it to receive the fertilized egg.

When the egg erupts from the follicle, its former home continues to grow and it secretes more estrogen and another hormone, progesterone, to the point that pituitary activity shuts down entirely. The body waits to see if the ejected egg will be fertilized.

In the absence of a pregnancy, the follicle withers. The endometrium, now denied the support, of its hormones, sloughs and bleeds, resulting in menstruation.

These first cycles initiate the fertile era. Ensuing menstrual cycles for the next forty or so years significantly influence a woman's entire life. Though modern methods of birth control have reduced the importance of the menstrual cycle, a woman's body will continue to be affected by the hormones that regulate the monthly period.

In addition to regulating her menstrual cycle, the hormone estrogen also has a beneficial effect on a woman's health and well-being, a fact she may not realize even when she suffers the effects of its deficiency. Few women would argue that all the phases of cyclic hormone activity are pleasant. And many women welcome the menopause—not only as a relief from monthly discomfort, but as a release from the fear of unwanted pregnancy.

But the menopause is rarely uneventful. And it is during this period that a woman who has taken the time to learn what it is all about appreciates for the first time the importance that estrogen has played in her life. Too often, however, women who are reluctant to admit they have an estrogen deficiency place the blame for all their problems on some other real or imagined illness. Take the case of Miss Bigby. Miss Bigby came to me fifteen years ago complaining of symptoms which she was sure were due to hypoglycemia or low blood sugar.

"For years," she announced on our first meeting, "I suffered from fainting spells, which the doctors in Baltimore diagnosed as everything from low blood pressure to 'the vapors.' Then I consulted a specialist here in New York City who told me I had hypoglycemia. He put me on a diet and I have been in perfect health ever since—until recently that is."

For over a year, she went on to explain, she had become increasingly unwell. Her hypoglycemic specialist had retired; so she had tried to cope on her own. But no matter how she adjusted and readjusted her diet, she got worse.

I asked her to describe her symptoms, which sounded suspiciously like those of the climacteric.

"It is as if there is no more central control system in my body. I am always hungry or thirsty, the little energy I have comes in inexplicable spurts, I am hot when I should be cool, my heart races when I am sitting still, I am wide awake when I need to sleep and drowsy when I have to work. My disposition is so unpredictable I am afraid to be with people, and my periods long ago lost any semblance of a cycle, and I could go on and on."

I gave Miss Bigby a thorough examination, which revealed that she had two problems: diabetes and an estrogen deficiency. Her *hypo*glycemia had been, as is frequently the case, a prelude to *hyper*glycemia, too much sugar in the blood. When she returned for the results of her tests I explained the problem to Miss Bigby.

"Whereas your pancreas had been secreting too much insulin, now it is not secreting enough. This accounts for many of your symptoms, but not all. Your body is also suffering from a loss of its normal estrogen supply. You should have been aware of this over a year ago when your cycles became irregular and the flushes and sweats started. The absence of any sort of period for six months should have been a warning to see a doctor."

"And now that I am here, what is your advice?" she asked in a voice that challenged, while her winning smile never wavered.

I thought it best to begin with the problem that had first brought her to my office, so I returned to the subject of her insulin deficiency.

"First," I began, "your pancreas is not secreting enough insulin to handle the carbohydrates in your diet. As healthy as your eating habits are, diet is simply not sufficient care. Insulin replacement therapy is the most effective treatment for diabetes, and for the sake of your health, you must be prepared to take injections for the rest of your life."

That settled, I went on with what I sensed would be the more difficult problem. "Second," I said, "you need estrogen."

"That I do not need," she answered, bobbing her head for emphasis.

"I disagree," I rejoined quickly. "You are proud that

you are a woman and utilize all your feminine attributes. The thing that made you female—your body and to some extent your mind—is estrogen. But now you are deficient in this essential element and your body and mind are reacting, just as they are reacting to your insulin deficiency."

"But I'm not interested in sex or childbearing. My life is full of other things."

"You might have the potential for a full life," I told her firmly, "but you may never realize it without an adequate supply of estrogen. I wouldn't expect you to walk out of here without demanding that I take steps to control your diabetes. And I'd think you foolish if you didn't insist on controlling your estrogen deficiency as well."

She sat for a moment, slowly running her fingers through her hair in a gesture of conciliatory surrender. "Whatever you think," she answered finally, accepting my decision but tendering me all responsibility for it.

It was a responsibility I was happy to take. She was fifty then, younger than average for the degenerative diseases that often develop with aging. Now, at sixty-five, Miss Bigby is still getting everything she can out of life and still on estrogen replacement therapy. On a recent office visit, I asked her if she thought she should stop it. Her answer was as direct as my instruction had been fifteen years earlier.

"No thanks. I tried that once—unintentionally. I overlooked taking my pills with me when I went to Europe for the summer. I felt so bad and got so blue I literally begged a doctor to prescribe them. Within a week I was water-skiing and exploring cathedrals. The only problem I had was deciding which gentlemen I would let stake me at the roulette table."

It is difficult to say in any specific case exactly what role estrogen deficiency plays in degenerative changes of the body. But there is little doubt that it can contribute to— even accelerate—the aging process. After years of one menstrual cycle following another, the ovaries atrophy. The amount of hormone they secrete becomes erratic— sometimes too much, but usually too little. The feedback relationship the ovaries have had with the pituitary at one end and the uterine lining at the other is disrupted.

With the onset of ovarian atrophy the pituitary is released from the inhibition placed on it by the high levels of estrogen present in the second half of a normal menstrual cycle. The pituitary starts secreting its follicle-stimulating hormone (FSH) as it has done for years. But now none of the thousands of follicles remaining in the ovaries responds. It secretes more and more, frantically trying to arouse the moribund ovaries. And it is this abnormal amount of FSH that irritates the autonomic, or involuntary, nervous system, producing the classic menopausal symptoms: hot flushes, sweats, and dizziness. The excess of FSH may also interfere with other basic autonomic functions such as digestion, circulation, and respiration.

In addition, the brain—its biochemistry perhaps altered by these hormonal imbalances—is affected, often creating emotional disruptions. The result is a confused conglomeration of symptoms, including palpitations, numbness and tingling of the skin, gas, abdominal pains, nausea and vomiting, constipation and diarrhea. When concentrated in a short period, all or some of these symptoms are known as the "menopausal crisis"; when stretched over a period of months or even years, the "menopausal syndrome." We shall be discussing these differences in more detail in the following chapter.

The menopause itself—the actual cessation of the menses—is not without its own drama. The monthly cycles may become highly irregular. A cycle may be skipped or identifiable only by slight spotting. Or the final series of menses may be profuse and prolonged.

Ideally, the last scene in this drama is an ovary too weak to produce menstruation but still strong enough to furnish a sustaining amount of estrogen. More frequently, however, the final act of ovarian atrophy is played out slowly over the rest of a woman's life, when the long-term results of estrogen deficiency become manifest. These are the "silent" symptoms of the climacteric. They occur in tissues and organs that degenerate slowly from the estrogen deficiency. Some of the changes may never become serious enough to cause trouble. Others may not attract attention until some irreparable damage has been done. Because these symptoms may occur long after the menopause, their cause-and-effect relationship to estrogen deficiency is not always recognized. To appreciate the importance of estrogen as a biochemical agent, it is only necessary to examine what goes wrong if there is not enough.

The organs of reproduction shrink and lose their tone. This is not important in the tubes and the uterus, which can serve no future purpose. But it is important in their supporting structures and in the vagina and external genitalia. When their supporting ligaments and muscles deteriorate, the uterus and adjoining bladder and rectum are no longer held firmly in position. They tend to "drop" in the pelvic cavity. This protrusion, or prolapse, is commonly referred to as a "hernia." Surgical correction is sometimes necessary but the condition itself may be avoided if the estrogen deficiency is treated.

The vagina loses its distensibility and moisture. Its external folds (the labia) become flaccid and withered. Shrinkage of the milk glands contributes to sagging of the breasts. The changes in the breasts as well as in the labia are further accentuated by the loss of elasticity and hydration that the skin in general suffers as a result of estrogen deficiency. The mucous membranes, as well as the skin, can lose stamina and efficiency. Those lining the nose especially may become weak and may result in some loss of smell.

A loss of smell may seem insignificant, and compared with the ill effects on the vagina, it is. I, for one, am relieved that we as a society have detached ourselves from the myth that sexual activity and reproduction are one and the same. And we've certainly come a long way from our former dictum against sex after menopause. It seems especially cruel that at the very moment when women no longer must worry about unwanted pregnancy, many develop vaginal discomfort that limits their future sexual fulfillment. One of my own case histories comes immediately to mind.

The woman was referred to me by an older physician, a colleague of many years. Now he was to be remarried, and he decided that both he and his bride-to-be should have a thorough physical. I had already examined him and found him to be in good health. His future bride, Mrs. Delacroix, looked neither younger nor older than her fifty-seven years. Though she was easy to be with, her warm personality demanded respect. Her inner security made her physically and personally more attractive. She had come to New York five years earlier as dean of women at a small college. The events of the three years prior to her move had virtually dictated a change. Her husband had died, her son had moved to Australia, her previous job had become a bore, and she had had the menopause. Such a climacteric would have defeated some women. But Mrs. Delacroix had taken it all in her stride.

"I am ashamed to say, Dr. Parrish," she began as we

met to discuss the findings of the examination, "that you are the first physician I have consulted in almost eight years, when I was going through the change of life. But that doctor found me to be in excellent health and assured me that the symptoms would soon pass. They did, and I have felt fit ever since."

"No complaints at all Mrs. Delacroix?" I asked in a tone intentionally meant to convey that I had reason to think otherwise.

"Nothing really," she answered, as she tried to think back over the preceding years. "Nothing more than some female complaints, which I considered natural."

"Like what?" I continued to probe.

"I suppose it can best be described," she began, "as a vaginal irritation. I've been using an ointment which soothes the burning and itching, but the condition has not improved. Several areas around the vaginal opening are now almost constantly raw."

"So I noted in my examination," I told her. "The condition is called 'atrophic vaginitis.' After the menopause, the vagina is denied its usual nourishment of estrogen. The cells become too weak to repair themselves. The protective mucus they normally secrete becomes scant. Aside from being a problem of lubrication, the pH of the vagina, which is usually acid, becomes alkaline. This promotes an overgrowth of the organisms normally present, and causes inflammation."

"Of course I'm worried about the inflammation, Dr. Parrish, but frankly it's the lack of lubrication I was most concerned about. I'm hoping to make the most of my new marriage. What can be done about it?"

"Two things. The first is the local application of a cream that contains cortisone and estrogen. The cortisone will reduce the inflammation, while the estrogen will revitalize the cells."

"And the second?" she asked quickly.

"Estrogen replacement therapy to correct the deficiency that has caused the problem. But I am prescribing it for more than this local condition," I continued, taking advantage of a symptomatic problem to make her appreciate the importance of other as yet "silent" possibilities.

"Your atrophied ovaries may not be furnishing some other cells with the hormones they need. As you may have been conditioned to do, you dismissed the menopause as a trivial moment. No attempt was made to compensate for this important change. But from the results of your Estrogen Index, I'd suspect that other long-term difficulties might be waiting in the wings."

"My Estrogen Index?" she repeated.

"It is also called a Maturation Index, and is used to determine the development of the cells that respond to estrogen. At the time of a vaginal examination cells are scraped from the wall and examined microscopically. The color the cells stain reflects the influence of estrogen on them. Years of study have resulted in an index that defines the influence as high, low, or moderate. It is a test like a PAP smear when cells taken from the cervix of the uterus are examined for cancerous change. Because the vaginal mucosa registers estrogen activity, the Estrogen Index is an important guide to a woman's hormonal status."

"I guess I don't need to tell you, Doctor, that if it hadn't been for my marriage to David, I probably would never have consulted a physician for the next ten years. Even then, I'd probably have settled for just the required blood test—and certainly never had anything like an Estrogen Index. You say I'll have no trouble with my atrophia—"

"*Atrophic vaginitis.* No more trouble at all, particularly once your estrogen regimen gets under way. If you'd waited those ten years, I might not have been able to be so positive. The mucous membranes might have been permanently damaged. That lovely complexion of yours might have suffered, too," I added.

"Well, Dr. Parrish," she said, "I can see you have a lot to teach me."

"And I plan to do so. We're going to start you with one intramuscular estrogen injection today—and then about one every two weeks for a month or two. I'll keep track of your Estrogen Index, and decide which of the oral estrogen tablets we'll switch you to. Estrogen has to be carefully regulated."

"How many methods of estrogen therapy are there?" she asked.

"Several. Some doctors maintain patients with monthly injections, like the one I'll give you today. A few use pellets that can be implanted in the skin and slowly release the estrogen over a period of about six months. Then there are tablets."

"How do these estrogens differ from one another?" she wanted to know.

"The three most common types are synthetic, semisynthetic, and natural. The synthetic type does not have the chemical structure of estrogen but has its biological activity. It is the cheapest to manufacture, but is frequently not well tolerated by the body. The semisynthetic estrogen is a chemical re-creation of the natural hormone that has been altered to make it more potent. It is better tolerated and is commonly used in birth control pills.

"Natural estrogens are extracted from the urine of pregnant mares. Their activity is not as sustained or as strong as the synthetic and semisynthetic estrogens, and for this reason they would not be effective in birth control. Furthermore, in acute cases of estrogen deficiency when a constant effect is needed, they might have to be given in divided doses during the day. But because they are natural, they cause fewer side effects.

"I consider them best for ERT. If a woman is going to take estrogen the rest of her life, constant activity is not needed, and because natural estrogens are comparable to the one her ovaries would produce, they are well tolerated.

"The final choice depends on the doctor's preference and the patient's acceptance. The important thing is that the woman always has an adequate supply of this vital body biochemical. Whatever product is chosen, estrogen therapy must always be titrated—evaluated and adjusted—according to the patient's need. During the menopause itself the amount and method of administration are different from the regimen chosen to maintain her the rest of her life.

"In your case, I would like to start you with injections to obtain the maximum effect quickly. Once that has been achieved, I can determine the basic amount of oral estrogen to be taken on a regular basis. Oral ERT is the most effective and practical method. The dosage will be just enough to correct the degree of deficiency, and uterine bleeding will be unlikely."

I wrote out a prescription for her hormone cream, then instructed my nurse to give her her first injection.

On my way home that evening I thought of Mrs. Delacroix. She was alert, realistic, pleasant, and involved with life. Dr. Phillips was indeed lucky to have found and won her. I had no idea what their previous relationship had been, but I sincerely hoped that my therapy for her vaginitis would be quickly effective. Marriages are difficult enough without starting them off with a sexual problem. I knew that her positive attitude would speed her recovery but I was sorry that the problem had developed. For though she concealed her concern, I was certain she was troubled about it.

What troubled me was *the fact* that it had developed. Had she been aware of the symptoms earlier, her atrophic vaginitis could have been avoided. But though there is a natural tendency to place blame, I did not try. I had seen too many of these cases. It could have been her fault or her doctor's fault; but the basic fault, I had learned, was with society's attitude toward menopause. It is not given the respect it deserves.

In the past few years the medical profession has begun to realize the full consequences of estrogen deficiency. The menopause, with or without symptoms, should put both the patient and the physician on guard that sooner or later specific changes are likely. If this warning is heeded, there is no need for the degenerative diseases of estrogen deficiency to become blatantly and painfully obvious. But the menopause quickly slips into the past. The importance of an estrogen deficiency may not be taken into consideration during routine examinations.

The regimen I prescribed for Mrs. Delacroix produced the results we wanted. Within a few months after she returned, radiant, from her honeymoon, it was determined that 1.25 mg. of natural conjugated estrogens every other day was the optimum dosage for her. As long as she remained on this she would not be troubled with atrophic vaginitis—or many of the other degenerative diseases that frequently accompany ovarian atrophy.

I have found this regimen—sometimes modified to three times a week—to be the best for the average estrogen deficient postmenopausal woman. Some need more than twice this amount, and some can manage on half. Sometimes after the years pass, the dosage has to be increased. But side effects are uncommon, which is reassuring to both the patient and to me.

In younger women, those who are still going through the menopause, I prefer to administer estrogen on a cyclic basis to mimic the normal menstrual cycle. Estrogen is given for "x" number of weeks, during the last of which progesterone is given along with it to facilitate the withdrawal bleeding. The length of these cycles can be adjusted for from one month (including the week for the withdrawal bleeding or "artificial menses") to four months.

The value of this therapy lies in preventing an overgrowth of the uterine lining, which the amount of estrogen (the body's supply complemented by that of the oral preparation) cannot support. The uterus is cleaned out at intervals and the likelihood of breakthrough bleeding is reduced.

Administering estrogen in monthly cycles is most valuable in instituting ERT. Using the Estrogen Index, the occurrence of side effects, the relief of symptoms and the amount of menstrual flow, a doctor can get a good idea of the dosage of estrogen any particular women needs to correct her impending or existing estrogen deficiency. But many women, once they know their menses no longer serve a purpose, are anxious to reduce its inconvenience to a minimum. So when the doctor is sure of the required dosage he can extend the cycles.

Later in the postmenopausal years cyclic therapy, but not ERT, can be discontinued. Then the amount of estrogen based on the predetermined total monthly need can be divided throughout the week. This interrupted therapy can insure the woman enough estrogen to prevent the disasters of a deficiency, but because sensitive organs are not constantly stimulated the possibility of untoward effects is virtually eliminated. This is the therapy I prefer for women like Mrs. Delacroix, who have passed through the years when their ovaries are undergoing their atrophy. As time passes, the dose might have to be increased because further atrophy of the ovaries or compensatory supplies from the adrenal glands may continue to dwindle and more is needed to prevent a deficiency.

To accept and understand ERT is essential for its success. A little misinformation, a lot of prejudice, and a bad experience can work to a woman's detriment.

Such was the case with Hanna Schmidt. Mrs. Schmidt, who was sixty-seven years old, had been a patient of mine for six years, ever since her own doctor had retired. Hers was a complicated history of disorders that focused on an inherently weak endocrine system.

She had had several pregnancies, but all had ended in miscarriages. When she was thirty, a cyst had been excised from her left breast, and at thirty-five she had had surgery to remove a cyst so large it had virtually destroyed her left ovary. Both, however, were benign.

About twelve years later, after a difficult menopause, she began complaining of back pain and increasing stiffness, which she attributed to arthritis. But X-rays indicated the beginnings of *osteoporosis*, a disease in which the bones begin to lose both strength and solidity—a condition aggravated by estrogen deficiency.

When Mrs. Schmidt first came to me, I tried to relieve some of her misery. But after two years of her perfunctorily rejecting all of my suggestions, I concluded that she was not interested in being treated. Fundamentally, she had little use for the medical profession or for medicines, aside from a passionate faith in "buffered aspirin" for her backache. She seemed to enjoy ill-health, accepting it as a sort of martyrdom. It was the basis of her relationships to others—including her physician.

Sometimes she came with a specific complaint, but basically my function was to reassure her, twice a year after a thorough physical, that she did not have high blood pressure, diabetes, or cancer.

I was happy to oblige and happy I found nothing further wrong with her, except an occasional borderline elevation in her blood pressure. I never failed, however, to remind her about her osteoporosis, which was getting progressively worse. The disabling condition was evident not only in her X-rays but also in her stooping shoulders and continuous complaints of low back pain.

Had she begun taking some form of estrogen years before, during her menopause, her osteoporosis might have been negligible. For the beneficial effects of estrogen are not limited to the body's surface—the skin and mucous membranes—but extend to the skeletal system as well.

Estrogen exerts an anticatabolic effect on bone metabolism. With age the parathyroid glands that control calcium metabolism seem to become unbalanced. They exact more calcium from the bone than they replace. And unfortunately it is not just a matter of not enough calcium, and other bone minerals, in the diet. It is a degenerative phenomenon. Estrogen helps counteract it, inhibiting, through the complex interrelationships of the endocrine system, the parathyroid hormone destruction of bone. In other words, bone is living tissue, being built and broken down through a complicated combination of metabolic process. Beginning in the climacteric, destruction (catabolism) surpasses anabolism (building up).

Of the four million people in the United States who suffer from osteoporosis, 80 percent are female. The disease begins soon after the ovaries start to decline and will affect the lives of one-quarter of all postmenopausal women. The bones most severely affected are usually those most important in weight bearing—the hipbone, the vertebrae, and the bones of the forearm. After years of neglect, the disease is responsible for what is known as the "widow's hump"—a hunched posture that makes any woman look decades older than her years. Osteoporosis is usually at fault with fractures of the hip, so common in older women. And estrogen is our best weapon with which to fight back.

In Mrs. Schmidt's case, I was convinced—from experience and medical literature—that estrogens were not harmful in a patient with her history of benign cysts of the reproductive organs. I ventured on several occasions my opinion that she should try a period of low-dose estrogen replacement therapy. Inevitably her response was a cold stare, a shake of the head, and the unqualified comment of "no hormones." So I abandoned my attempt. But fate intervened to make the point that I had been unable to.

Hanna Schmidt fell and broke her wrist. It was not a hard fall. Bending over to pick up a thread on the rug, she lost her balance. As she broke her tumble with the palm of her hand, she heard the bones crack. I referred her immediately to an orthopedic specialist who, in view of the condition of her bones, was surprised that the fracture was not more severe. He did, however, have serious doubts about the speed and ability of the bones to knit properly.

Three days after her accident, she was in my office, looking more pathetic than ever with a black sling to support the heavy cast on her arm. She had come because copious amounts of buffered aspirin had done next to nothing to soothe the pain in her wrist, nor had the prescription the orthopedist had given her. She could not sleep, and during the day all she was able to do was pray the throbbing would stop. She almost pleaded for something to stop the pain.

I felt sorry for her, but intuitively something told me to attack this vulnerability instead of consoling her.

"Of course, Mrs. Schmidt, I will give you something to relieve the pain as well as something to help you sleep. But remember these only alleviate the symptoms, they do not eliminate the cause. Both strong analgesics and hypnotics are invaluable in times of acute distress. But they are no substitutes for medicines that correct the basic problem. I am much more worried about the state of your skeletal system and the recovery power of your bone metabolism. You have severe osteoporosis; your bones have lost a lot of mineral substance and are very brittle."

"I cannot help that," she answered defensively. "That is my constitution."

"You *can* help yourself," I countered emphatically. "First, your diet is deficient in many of the elements that the bone needs to keep regenerating itself, particularly protein and calcium. You need more meat and less potatoes. Skimmed milk will take care of some of the calcium deficiency, but not all. I would also recommend a calcium tablet that contains fluorine and other trace minerals and bone needs as well as vitamin D, which is necessary for the absorption and utilization of the calcium."

To my surprise, she took the prescription I handed her without objection, and I seized the opportunity to drive home my point. "Although these nutrients can help curb abnormal bone resorption," I continued, "they do not cure osteoporosis. You should be taking estrogen."

Then I got the reaction I had anticipated. "I'm not taking any of that. It causes cancer."

"Mrs. Schmidt, I consider you an informed woman, and in my opinion, an informed patient is the best patient. I'm sure you know that in medicine,perhaps more than in any other field, we have to deal with both facts and circumstances and adapt them to highly individualized problems. Considering your case in the light of all available information, I believe that supplemental estrogen is indicated."

"Are you saying there is no risk?" she asked.

"Any medicine or form of treatment has some element of risk," I replied. "This must be weighed against the potential benefits. It is not impossible for a woman of your age to develop cancer of the breast or uterus, but you, as an individual, are far more likely to have serious, perhaps grave problems from complications of osteoporosis."

"But if there is a risk, Doctor, why take a chance—no matter how small it may be?"

"Because I am treating you as a person—not as a disease. You have come for your checkups regularly for years, and I know you'll continue to do so. I feel certain that you will follow my directions for the use of your estrogen, and not exceed the prescribed dosage. I know, too, that you will cooperate when I feel it is necessary to do an endometrial biopsy—that is to check for any unanticipated change in the cells lining your womb. No doctor wants to prescribe *any* medication unless it is necessary, and I have no doubt you need these pills."

"But cancer! Just the idea is frightening.!"

"I agree, but it has been fifteen years since your menopause, these tissues have probably shrunk to the point where there would be little response, let alone the growth of a malignancy, to a limited dose of estrogen."

I paused a moment for emphasis. "In the practice of medicine a doctor has to make a decision. That is one of the things he is paid for—his judgment. Using his experience, his knowledge of a particular patient, and the pros and cons of a particular therapy, he must decide whether or not its benefits outweigh its possible harm. Sometimes he may want to do further studies or get the opinion of another doctor. Then he presents his recommendations to the patient.

"For you I strongly recommend estrogen. Only two months ago your Index showed *no* estrogen influence. But if you are uneasy, I will arrange for any further tests or consultations you want. They will confirm that you have no latent cancer. On the other hand, it has already been confirmed that you have osteoporosis, which is now interfering with the proper healing of your fracture. This disease demands estrogen therapy to correct a defect in your bone metabolism."

I paused. "But the decision is up to you. I can only give you the benefit of my knowledge and experience. It is your life."

Mrs. Schmidt looked thoughtful for a moment, then responded matter-of-factly, "I will take it for a few months. Then we will see." She paused, "When will they take the cast off?"

"As soon as possible. Immobilization and inactivity aggravate the healing process, especially in the presence of osteoporosis."

In three months she came back to the office. The cast had been off for several weeks, and though her wrist had limited mobility there was no deformity.

"The doctor is very pleased," she said proudly. "He even seems surprised at my progress. And I, myself, can see, judging from those exercises he prescribed, a little improvement every day."

I do not know if she recognized it, but I also noted that her psychological attitude was more positive and I felt that physically she was stronger. Her semiannual examination, due in another month, would give me some concrete evidence for comparison. And before she left, she gave me another reason to feel I would be satisfied with those findings.

"Skimmed milk is not so bad," she said. "And both my husband and I have found out that a rare steak and a big, fresh salad make a rather pleasant evening meal."

She had listened, had a new experience, learned, and I felt sure, profited. The proverbial best teacher, experience, can only come with living. The experience of aging is best utilized to make each future year a step forward. There has not yet been found—and probably never will be—a method of stopping the progressive physical changes in our body. But the dramatic benefits of ERT can slow some of those changes and make the later years a time of ongoing fulfillment and involvement in life.

"Doctor, I'm Falling Apart"

The Menopausal Crisis and Syndrome

As we have seen, every middle-aged woman is subjected to certain biological changes. And those changes center around the one constant factor of the climacteric—the menopause. Some women breeze through it with little discomfort; others may experience varying degrees of distress.

The manner in which the ovaries abandon their usual function strongly influences the course of the menopause. If they atrophy slowly, if the organs they influence are not hypersensitive, and if they continue to supply a sustaining amount of estrogen, symptoms are insignificant. But if their decline is erratic, if the end organs overreact to the hormonal imbalance, and if the estrogen supply becomes markedly deficient, problems are inevitable. Symptomatic menopauses can be generally divided into those in which the symptoms are moderate and prolonged, a *menopausal syndrome*, and those in which they are of briefer duration but more severe, a *menopausal crisis*.

30

Whether the symptoms of a menopausal crisis are primarily physical or psychological, their manifestation is one of acute distress. Such was the case with a recent patient, Mrs. De Marina. She was about fifty years old, alert, and very sophisticated. Her natural features were accentuated by careful grooming and tasteful, expensive clothes. On her first visit, she had calmly extended her hand, eased into the chair and then suddenly thrown her arms into the air and blurted out:

"Doctor, I'm falling apart! Please help me."

I was a little taken aback since she seemed to be in no acute discomfort.

"Don't try to ask me what's wrong because everything is," she sputtered.

"Whatever is bothering you," I said, "had to start at some point with some symptom or sign."

"Not necessarily," she said, sitting so far forward that I was afraid she would slip off the chair. "It could have begun three months, or three weeks, or three days ago. It was first a little thing here, a little thing there; then in the last few days all the little things have come together. I can't take it any longer. I feel like Humpty Dumpty, in a hundred pieces."

Evidently somewhat relieved by her outburst, she settled back into the chair, and then continued emphatically, "I'm certain no woman has had so many things go wrong with her all at once. You must do something. This is a terrible way to live."

"So far you have spoken only in general terms," I responded matter-of-factly so as not to increase her hysteria. "But if I am going to be of help, we must get down to some specifics. I have the feeling that you have always been healthy, unaccustomed to illness. So suddenly being besieged by all these problems is understandably disturbing."

She relaxed a bit with the satisfaction that she was not going to be ignored.

"Let's try to find a beginning somewhere," I suggested.

"I'll try," she said. "You're right; I've always had a healthy body that served me well, rarely complaining. I don't think I have abused it, but in general I have eaten what I liked, never had to worry about my weight, worked and played the way I pleased, was not uncomfortable in drafty corners others avoided, ignored colds and backaches, skied, climbed mountains, swam, and never suffered from sinus trouble or indigestion or any of those irksome things.

"I had two children as easily as a cat has kittens. Furthermore, I never had any so-called female problems. Then suddenly four months ago my periods became unpredictable and confusing. Everyone says we are having a mild November. But for me it's hot—then cold—then warm—then wet. I have never perspired before in my life unless I did a lot of exercise. Now sometimes, just as I finish something as easy as putting on my makeup, my whole forehead is drenched with sweat.

"I go to bed perfectly comfortable, finally doze off, and then wake up suffocating under nothing more than a light blanket. I open the windows, go back to bed, but in a few hours I wake shivering with cold perspiration. It's a nightmare.

"Daytime is no different—it's too hot or too cold. I've had the superintendent up at least a dozen times, but he says there's nothing wrong with the thermostat."

"It seems to be that the problem is with your body's thermostat," I ventured.

"I don't care whose it is, I just want it fixed. Then maybe I can get a good night's rest."

"Do you have difficulty going to sleep?"

"Yes, in spite of the fact that I'm tired all the time. The whole routine of my life, as well as my sleeping pattern, has changed, and I can't get used to it. I never know what to expect; I never know how I am going to feel. I don't know whether I want to be alone or with people. And I know people don't want to be with me. The slightest thing can make me erupt, fly into a tantrum. But if I am alone I get depressed."

Half angry, half bewildered, Mrs. De Marina looked at me.

"Dr. Parrish, am I going crazy?"

"No," I said. "Your body has apparently been thrown off balance; some of its functions have lost their normal rhythm. And no doubt this has upset you emotionally."

"But it has never happened before! Why all of a sudden now?"

"It would be wrong for me to speak with any certainty after only hearing this brief history. However, I can make an educated guess.

"As I am sure you know, nature limits the years of a woman's fertility. To effect this, some biological programming we don't understand inhibits the ovaries from producing ova and they begin to atrophy. They stop serving a useful purpose long before the rest of a woman does. As they atrophy, they no longer secrete the hormones which have been influencing and regulating her fertility, things such as the menstrual cycle."

"I hope you are trying to tell me I have reached my menopause; I'm ready. But why must my ovaries instigate all this turmoil? If they are finished with what they are supposed to do, they should dry up and leave me alone."

"They will, sooner or later. Sometimes they stop functioning abruptly without causing any trouble or their decline is gradual and any symptoms are insignificant. Sometimes their atrophy springs open a Pandora's box. But usually their atrophy is capricious—periods of overactivity and underactivity are interspersed with normal periods, until finally the ovaries are too weak to have any effect."

I continued my explanation because I wanted to put her as much at ease as possible before I examined her.

"When the ovaries atrophy, they not only stop producing eggs, they stop secreting their hormones. Your body has to adjust. Sometimes this presents no problem, especially if some ovarian tissue continues to function and provides a residual supply of estrogen. On the other hand, a deficiency of estrogen can disrupt important physiologic functions that may even affect how long you live.

"So thinking positively, if my presumptive diagnosis is correct, your symptoms can be considered cries for help. Women whose menopause is uncomplicated may not be as lucky. They have no disturbing symptoms that motivate them to find out if their body is deficient in estrogen."

"I'd have been quite satisfied if I had just suddenly quit menstruating and been spared any SOS."

"That's a natural, but frequently unfortunate, attitude. Most women can ignore a few hot flashes. And they consider a few days of irritability a small price to pay for an easy menopause. But no woman should be satisfied about a cessation of her menses until she had consulted her doctor. After all, the end of the menstrual cycle, the actual menopause, is a sign that something in her body has changed. It is her duty to find out as exactly as possible what has happened."

Mrs. De Marina seemed more relaxed, though still concerned. "Tell me what causes these hot flashes, Doctor. I'm embarrassed to go shopping; perspiration drops on things I'm looking at. Or if I'm lunching with a friend, it can even drop into my food. Something has to be terribly wrong." 1900441

"Something is wrong; but whether or not it is abnormal is a question medicine hasn't settled yet. Until recently it was generally accepted that such turmoil at the time of the change of life was to be expected. Then the sex hormones were discovered and science learned how the ovaries were able to affect other parts of the body. When the ovaries no longer send out these sex hormones, the body reacts. Some of the effects are noticed immediately; some, actually more serious, may not be noted for years."

I thought her attention was flagging, so I came back to her immediate problem. "The hot flashes you are having now are one of the first symptoms of ovarian decline. They can be considered 'natural' but not necessarily 'normal.' An important gland, the pituitary, which masterminds the endocrine system, is not getting regular reports from the ovaries. So it sends out its own messengers to try to get them to function. But the ovaries are not capable of responding as they should. The pituitary then sends out more stimulating hormones. And it is an excess of these hormones that causes the flushes and sweats. It disrupts certain mechanisms that regulate the body temperature."

I saw that I had Mrs. De Marina's attention again. "Not only do the flushes and the sweats vary in duration, they vary in frequency and severity. They also vary from woman to woman. Typically the flush is sudden and unpredictable in onset, starting above the waist and spreading up the chest and back to the neck and face. Isolated patches at other sites may occur, but the entire body is not involved. Accompanying the glow of the flush is a sensation of warmth. This is usually, but not necessarily, followed by sweating, particularly of the forehead and upper chest. Then the evaporation of the perspiration produces a feeling of chilliness.

"This is the reason you never seem to be able to stabilize a comfortable temperature. The imbalance of hormones suddenly triggers the blood vessels, especially those close to the surface, to dilate. It's not understood exactly why or how. This same disorder, which is called a vasomotor disturbance, may alter other biological functions, possibly the circulation in the brain, which could explain episodes of dizziness. Certainly the experience of vasomotor flushing and sweating affects the peace of mind.

"But your thermostat will behave more appropriately when your pituitary is convinced your ovaries have retired permanently or we have satisfied its concern about them with estrogen replacement therapy."

"What's that?" she asked with vague interest.

"Exactly what it says—administering this hormone in a sufficient amount to maintain one's normal health and well-being." I signaled my nurse, who took Mrs. De Marina into the examining room. I wanted to give her a complete physical to determine the general state of her health and also to determine how her ovaries were functioning. I also wanted to get an Estrogen Index.

When we had returned to my office I outlined and explained the therapy I intended to prescribe. Since she was unaccustomed to taking medication, I was specific in my directions. I prescribed a low dosage tranquilizer. She was to take one on arising and one at six-hour intervals until she was ready for bed. If she was unable to sleep, she was to take, instead of a sleeping pill, one or two more tranquilizers. Having limited the number to be dispensed by the pharmacist, I could reassure her that there was no possibility of overdosage. I knew she inherently objected to "taking pills," but experience had taught me that relieving anxiety and insuring adequate sleep expedited the treatment of these cases.

I also prescribed estrogen. There was little doubt that her symptoms were due—directly or indirectly—to ovarian dysfunction. Her history was classic—a middle-aged woman whose menses are variable in time and amount of flow and who experiences unpredictable episodes of flushing and sweating. These vasomotor phenomena and menstrual irregularities are primary symptoms because they can be directly related to the hormonal imbalance that results from the erratic decline of her ovaries.

The dizziness that Mrs. De Marina also complained of was probably another vasomotor symptom. But like her unpredictable changes of mood its cause could have been psychological as well as hormonal. Any physician who has seen a woman through the climacteric is well aware that it is a condition in which the mind and body are intimately involved. As a result, symptoms are innumerable.

There are, however, certain symptoms, which though not typical are not infrequent: peculiar sensations in the skin; digestive disturbances such as gas, abdominal pains, nausea and vomiting, constipation and diarrhea; respiratory difficulties; headaches; fatigue; insomnia; loss of appetite; anxiety, and depression. Whether these are physical or psychological will be discussed later. But one thing is certain. The climacteric is characterized by unpredictable changes in physical and mental functions that have for too long been taken for granted.

Circumstances make these years a period that necessitates a review of the past, an assessment of the present, and a plan for the future. Virtually every aspect of a woman's life is subject to change. One may be for the worse; another for the better. Her mind and body may support her completely; or one or the other, and

sometimes both, may fail her. Their functioning deter-
mines how she manages her course through these years
and how she copes with the problems presented her.

Since a wide variety of factors influence the
symptomatology of the menopause, its manifestation can
be as individual as the faces of the women who pass
through it. It is virtually impossible to predict how any
particular woman will tolerate the menopause. The
human element cannot be ignored. Though usually the
severity of symptoms is directly related to a woman's basic
emotional stability, strong women can become weak and
weak women strong. It has been my experience that the
reaction of most is markedly affected by fear—fear of the
unknown.

Certainly fear complicated the case of Mrs. De Marina,
whose fright required more attention than her hormonal
disorder. Since the onset of her menopause had been
sudden, she had had little time to adjust to the changes in
her physiology. She became acutely aware of her body,
and the slightest alteration of an expected function could
throw her into a tailspin. I prescribed estrogen for
specific therapy, tranquilizers as symptomatic therapy,
but a sympathetic ear was the most effective medicine
during the early days of her treatment.

I had to reassure her time and again that she was not
suffering from some fatal disease and that each day of
therapy brought her closer to a resolution of her crisis.
Absorbed as she was in her own distress, she found it
difficult to believe that other women had been similarly
afflicted. She became almost obsessed. A pervasive
preoccupation with changes introduced by the climacteric is not rare, but it is usually focused on psychological
aspects of age and aging. Mrs. De Marina's was rooted in
her physical symptoms.

No doubt there was an emotional overlay as well. She

had recently gone through a divorce, which was still having its repercussions. Except for the death of a spouse, there is no greater stress in mid-life than divorce. Separation and divorce are becoming increasingly important factors that color and complicate the climacteric. Physically and mentally, Mrs. De Marina probably would not have been so brittle at the time of her ovarian decline had she had the support of an understanding husband. But she did not, and her symptoms seemed to multiply rather than dissipate. Yet she could not be called a hypochondriac because there was good cause for many of her complaints.

I knew that she was uncomfortable but there was no cause for undue alarm. No matter how severe menopausal symptomatology might be, experience has convinced me that it can be controlled. What I had to do was convince her and get her cooperation in taking the prescribed medications. I also wanted her to be with other people, and gave my hearty approval when she decided to spend a holiday with her family. The holiday meal was good therapy and lifted her mood—perhaps too much.

Shortly thereafter, her two daughters came to spend a weekend. Mrs. De Marina was anxious that they not discover that she was ill, and she discontinued her tranquilizers without consulting me. I do not mind patients adjusting the dosage of certain medications but not until they are familiar with the use and need of that medication in their particular case.

Mrs. De Marina was not prepared. The medicine had not had time to establish by itself or give her the opportunity to establish emotional equanimity. And when she neglected to take her medication she set the stage for the exact scene she wanted to avoid. After a night of only a few hours' sleep, she was so irritable and peculiar that her daughters were alarmed. Frantically she took her tranquilizers, one too many as a matter of fact. She became drowsy and her behavior slowed, something she did not want her daughters to notice. But they did, and she had to tell them about her condition. Intellectually she intended to paint an optimistic picture, but she succeeded in portraying gloom and alarming her daughters—which, unconsciously, was probably what she wanted to do.

After this initial attempt at self-treatment, however, Mrs. De Marina followed my directions. The symptoms of her menopausal crisis did not disappear overnight. Her body thermostat, menstrual flow, and mood continued erratic for several weeks. But the exacerbations became less frequent and less severe, and she became less disturbed by them. She became more realistic, not being deceived by periods of good days only to be depressed when something went awry. One day about three weeks after she had originally come to see me, she said: "Things have been relatively quiet, but this horror is by no means over. The Furies are still capable of a resounding attack. Even on my best days I feel some sort of vague threat. I can't describe it, but it is as if my body as well as my mind were registering the effects of some unusual changes. I don't like it, but it keeps me on my toes. When this feeling is particularly strong, I know I must double my efforts at distracting my thoughts and I don't try to postpone taking a tranquilizer. Sometimes I even want to take more estrogen, but I know it won't do any good. You have been specific about that. I only wish that the ERT would hurry and reestablish my old hormonal status quo."

The fact that she came to this acceptance soon after treatment was started (actually sooner than I expected her to), probably contributed to her speedy recovery. She was no longer the hysterical woman who had first come

into my office, and within a few months she had regained
the equilibrium she feared she had lost forever.

Of course, not all women have so dramatic a time as Mrs.
De Marina. Aside from the many women who sail
through the change with hardly a problem, there are
those whose symptoms play hide-and-seek over a period
of time. For months—even years—a symptom will come
and go, be replaced by another, seemingly unrelated
problem, until suddenly they return in tandem, more
serious than ever.

This is the situation I have referred to as the
menopausal syndrome. The syndrome is differentiated
from the menopausal crisis mainly by its time factor.
Whereas the crisis generally appears as a mass of
symptoms, completely disrupting a woman's physical
and emotional health, the syndrome is a much sneakier
phenomenon. A symptom here, a symptom there, may
allow a woman a feeling of false security. The individual
symptoms, she reasons, may not be acute enough to
consult a physician. And, in the absence of any real
knowledge of the menopause and its patterns, the un-
wary victim fails to realize that her various ailments are
related at all.

"It's just old age," Rose Kent kept telling herself—and
presumably would have gone on doing so if her case had
not been brought to my attention by a friend who recognized her "old age" for what it really was.

Rose Kent had been referred to me by Doris Wieder, a
faithful patient of mine for many years. Doris and I had
collaborated on her mild menopausal crisis, and her
careful attention to her slight estrogen deficiency had
kept her trouble free ever since. So I was naturally
surprised when she phoned my office one afternoon

asking if headaches and stomach trouble could have anything to do with the menopause.

My answer was an equivocal "yes." But I was quick to reassure her that her estrogen regimen should prevent any such symptoms. "Perhaps," I told her, "you've been under some sort of strain."

"Oh, Dr. Parrish," she answered, "I couldn't be better. It's my husband's secretary I'm worried about. Rose has been with Harold for almost twenty years now, and he couldn't live without her. And to tell you the truth I don't think I could either. She always sees to it that Harold's home on time if we have any evening plans, she always lets me know what to pack for him when he has to go away, she even helps me out when my checkbook gets messed up."

Then she went on to describe some of the problems Rose Kent had been experiencing. For about a year, she had been troubled with what she called migraine headaches. "Dr. Parrish," Doris continued, "I don't think she's been to a doctor in twenty years, and if I can't understand what makes a headache 'migraine,' I don't see how she can!"

I agreed that the term "migraine" is thrown about rather loosely. "Maybe Mrs. Kent is under pressure. Is Harold working her too hard?"

"It's *Miss* Kent," Doris corrected me, "and if Harold is working her too hard I'll kill him. I'd like to think that tension was all that's wrong, Doctor—I really would. Rose lives in the same apartment building as her mother, you see, with the mother pretty well up in years. And I know the pressure is taking its toll. But lately she's also been complaining of recurrent bouts of nausea."

"Well, I think you've solved your own mystery, Doris. The woman is obviously anxious—and probably depressed at the way she takes out her anxiety on her mother. Tension headaches, stomach trouble, it adds up fairly well, don't you think?"

"Well, she told me the other night she was having some 'female troubles.' She wouldn't talk about it any further—she was positively whispering the words, what little I could get out of her. Could it be the menopause, Doctor—all spread out like that?"

"Possibly. The menopause, if you remember, is literally a onetime event, but the symptoms of the estrogen deficiency that cause it can go on for months—even years—before and after it."

"Would you see her, Dr. Parrish?" she asked.

"Of course. Have her phone for an appointment."

Doris paused for a moment. "She'll never do it, I'm afraid."

I leveled with her. "Doris, look. I can't drag the woman in off the street; she has to walk in that door on her own. Get Harold to talk her into it. He can phone my secretary and set up a day and time. After all the appointments she's made for him—and made him keep—he can make one for her."

"I'll get her there, Doctor. Thank you."

I didn't have much time that afternoon to think further about Rose Kent, but Doris Wieder must have turned her convincing voice to Miss Kent immediately. Two days later Rose Kent was waiting in my office as I walked in the door.

From my patient's extravagant praise, I suppose I must have been expecting a combination Amazon and majordomo. Instead, I found a tiny, fragile woman not more than an inch over five feet tall, with a sweet musical voice.

Doris Wieder was right about one thing: Miss Kent had not had a check-up in twenty years. She was right about another, too: Rose did have the menopause—or, more correctly, a scattered collection of symptoms all related to the decline of her ovaries—and all as on-again-off-again as the erratic menstrual flow she hesitantly described. In other words, she was suffering from a menopausal syndrome.

Rose declined the use of any short-term tranquilizers to relieve her irritability, but she was practically overjoyed at the thought that the estrogen therapy I prescribed would bring her menstrual cycle into a regular pattern. "All my life I've never known when to expect my periods," she told me, "and, of course, in the last year they've become an absolute mystery."

I explained to her that the twenty-one days of daily estrogen with the addition of progesterone the last five days, followed by a week off the hormones, should produce a regular flow. I often keep patients on a regular monthly cycle at first, the better to monitor their response to the hormone dosages. After that, I usually recommend stopping the estrogen—and thereby stimulating bleeding—only three or four times a year. This reduces the possibility of unexpected (or "breakthrough") bleeding, without the bother of a monthly flow.

Rose Kent, however, had ideas of her own. As I explained the estrogen/progesterone mechanism, and its relation to menstruation, I noticed a strange look in her eye. "Am I going too fast, Miss Kent?" I asked.

"No, Doctor, not at all. I was just wondering—well, does it hurt to continue periods for a few years after one's time is up?"

"Ordinarily, not at all. Why do you ask?"

"Because I think I'd like to keep them for a while. . . ."

We didn't speak any further of it at the time, but I eventually came to feel that Rose found considerable reassurance in the continuation of a "natural" menses.

Perhaps it made her feel younger, or perhaps she took some real delight, for the first time in her life, in having regular, dependable periods. However, I was happy to comply with her wishes—and she continues on a monthly cycle to this day.

Fortunately, no permanent deterioration had resulted from Rose Kent's neglect of her symptoms. A low dosage of supplemental estrogen was sufficient to reduce her tension, end her sporadic bleeding, and allow her to put back some of the weight she'd lost.

She continued to consult me once a month, at first, while we adjusted her estrogen dosage, then three times a year. She is a changed woman, cheerful, vigorous, and energetic. She never misses an appointment, and never misses a chance to thank me for what she terms— probably quite rightly—her revitalization.

Some twenty-five years of experience has convinced me that with few exceptions estrogen replacement therapy can calm the chaos created by the onset of the menopause—both in crisis situations like that of Mrs. De Marina and in more drawn-out cases, like Rose Kent's. This being so, it's only natural to wonder why *all* women are not maintained on hormones from the onset of the menopause until the death.

The answer is multifaceted. Some women, as I have noted, continue to produce residual hormones sufficient to ward off the ill effects of estrogen deficiency. They don't need, and shouldn't have, ERT.

And then there is the cancer controversy. It has existed and complicated ERT since hormones were discovered. Study after important study dispels this fear. But some isolated reports (based more on statistics than clinical evidence) have cast a shadow of a doubt on the subject. No matter how circumstantial their evidence, it cannot be ignored. Though I do not believe estrogens cause cancer,

I respect these reports because they make me and my patients aware that we are dealing with an important biochemical, which for all of its benefits, carries, as does any other medication, a potential risk.

But that is what the practice of medicine is all about. The prescription of hormones, just like tranquilizers and antibiotics, must be individualized. It is a matter of need versus danger. And I can think of no more appropriate example of individualizing therapy than "the pill."

It too is based on the pharmacologic activity of estrogen. The side effects are well known—water retention, weight gain, blood clots, nausea, yeast infections. But so are the benefits, which include avoiding the unhappiness of an unwanted pregnancy or the disabilities of—even death from—childbearing. But the decision to use or reject it rests with the woman and her physician. This is especially true in the later years of childbearing when the pill may become that "extra" factor that can precipitate a possible cardiovascular accident.

Though the use of estrogen is different in ERT—to correct a physiologic deficiency rather than create an abnormal amount to suppress ovulation—it is essential that it too be regulated and monitored. This applies not only to adjusting the dosage from woman to woman but also adjusting it to her needs in various stages of her menopausal and postmenopausal years. If a woman is to enjoy the benefits of ERT, then both she and her doctor must commit themselves to the practical vigilance which is the hallmark of good medicine.

There is little controvesy about ERT during a menopausal crisis or syndrome. Then its benefits are obvious. But since these conditions are self-limiting, once the body has adjusted to the ovarian atrophy, and the acute symptoms of estrogen deficiency have passed, the value of continued ERT comes into question. It is no longer a "medicine" to control disturbing symptomatology, but has become a preventive regimen to protect against the possible damages of a prolonged deficiency. It is this prolonged ERT that is criticized by some as being potentially hazardous.

Having been convinced of the value of continued ERT in women who are deficient in their natural supply, my primary concern is not the fear that it will create a cancer but that unexpected uterine bleeding will disrupt the patient's peace of mind. Bleeding is the first sign of abnormal changes in the uterine lining; and, like the reports that estrogen causes cancer, it cannot be ignored. But the likelihood of untoward or unwanted effects from estrogen supplementation can be virtually eliminated if the ERT is regulated and the endometrium examined periodically. Every precaution should be taken to ascertain that the amount of estrogen supplied is enough to keep the cells from atrophying but not so much that they overgrow. Giving the estrogen in cycles that are terminated every few months by the addition of progesterone, the secondary female hormone, produces a medical curettage that cleans out the womb. How frequently this should be done must be based on a reconciliation between the doctor and patient, with his knowledge taking precedence over the inconvenience of the "menstrual" flow.

Cyclic therapy every month or two is my recommendation for the critical years of the menopause. As the years pass, the length of the cycles can be extended. And once well into the postmenopausal years when a woman's natural supply of estrogen has stabilized and the amount of supplemental estrogen needed to prevent a deficiency has been determined, the estrogen can be given in interrupted doses two to four times a week with a medical curettage only once or twice a year.

My preference for ERT is natural conjugated estrogens, a choice favored by practicing physicians as well as scientific investigators. Not only has it been demonstrated over the last thirty years to have special benefits, such as providing a sense of well-being; it has the advantage of a limited period of activity, rarely extended over twenty-four hours. This negates its efficacy as an estrogen for birth control but enhances its value in supplying the limited needs of estrogen-deficient cells.

No woman need suffer the symptoms of the menopause. Whether they are crystallized into a crisis or protracted over a period of months or even years, modern medicine is able to offer relief.

There cannot, however, be any set regimen, because the turmoil at this time of life is not limited to ovarian decline. The menopause is but one aspect of the climacteric. Other changes are taking place in a woman's body and in her life. Changes in her relationship and obligation toward her husband, her family, her friends, her work, and herself can create other symptoms that demand attention. But she *can* get specific relief from the many symptoms that respond to estrogen replacement therapy. In this respect she is more fortunate than her male counterpart. There is no "miracle" hormone to relieve the problems of his middle years. But there has been some progress in that direction, if only that the medical profession is becoming increasingly aware of those problems and is reaching for some solutions.

"Something Seems to Be Wrong"

The Male Climacteric

Men also undergo certain psychological and physiological changes in mid-life. Unfortunately, the male does not have such an obvious signal as the menopause to warn him that the time of change is at hand. Therefore, his climacteric is more difficult to define in terms of age as well as pattern. It can be recognized anywhere between the late thirties and late sixties, but there is no focal point around which symptoms crystallize into a condition that can be diagnosed easily. In the absence of specific symptoms, men seldom seek the medical help they need. A thorough examination could detect and even deter some of the biological problems and maladjustments in progress, but they attract little attention until a heart attack or an acute depression turns the climacteric from a period of transitional stress into a crisis.

It was the former that brought Ronald Boyles, a long-time patient, in for his annual physical four months early. Knowing him to be a precise man, befitting an executive of a computer programming company, I was puzzled.

"Dr. Parrish," Mr. Boyles said, "I want as thorough an examination as you can give me. Something serious seems to be wrong with me; my body and even, I'm afraid to say, my mind."

He went on to explain that shortly after his last checkup eight months earlier, he had noticed that his energy level was flagging. Getting up in the morning had become a chore, and he could hardly wait to get home in the evening, though the piles of unfinished paper work at the office had begun to accumulate alarmingly. Never a man given to hearty laughter and indiscriminate enthusiasm, he now found he had lost even his gentle good humor. He was dour, easily irritated, and where once a single drink was enough to relax him, he now caught himself drinking more than a few. He recognized that his drinking was not to help express his good nature, but rather, to suppress his bad feelings.

Many problems had contributed to this negative state of mind; some of them he accepted as real, others he supposed were imagined or magnified. First, his eldest son had dropped out of college—for the third time. Second, his wife seemed more interested in local politics than in him. Meanwhile, the effect of the national recession had been felt in his own company. Salary increases and promotions were limited that year, and he no longer felt the security he once had in his job. This insecurity was further aggravated by his administration of his firm's lobbying expenses. He had handled the funds wisely, he felt, and honestly, but the current trend of exposing and investigating political improprieties had combined with his already unstable emotional state to create a psychological condition bordering on paranoia.

Although he knew that his economic situation was sound, he found himself constantly mulling over past mistakes and blaming himself for lack of foresight. At night, after he had submerged his hostility toward his wife for indifferently falling into a sound sleep while he lay awake brooding, he formulated plans to overcome the inertia he felt. But he never translated his plans into actions. His sense of insecurity and helplessness had grown into anxiety and depression, and a vicious cycle resulted: anxiety fostered indecision; inaction deepened depression. He was frightened—frightened that his life had been checkmated by circumstances beyond his control.

Then he turned his fear toward his physical condition. At first he had dismissed his fatigue as overwork. But its persistence, even after a long restful July weekend, worried him. The worry blossomed into full-fledged anxiety as he suffered inexplicable bouts of gas and constipation, acid indigestion, headaches, shortness of breath, a tender elbow, and blurred vision. He also had to urinate frequently, sometimes with an urgency he thought he could not control.

He was particularly disconcerted by his awareness of drafts, feeling chilled in his shoulders on a relatively balmy July evening. And when one of his children remarked that he was wearing wool socks with his bedroom slippers, he flew into a rage. He suddenly felt old.

He tried to analyze what he was doing wrong, what food and drink were bad for him, how many hours of sleep his body needed. He quit smoking, gave up red wines and bourbon, avoided spices, onions, and late meals, and had coffee only in the morning. Saturdays were devoted to necessary chores, and Sundays to enjoyment, accentuating outdoor activities. His hacking cough disappeared along with some of his excess stomach acidity and he did not seem to tire as quickly. He began to feel better.

Then late in August, as he was enjoying a beer after a

fast set of tennis, his heart seemed to veer out of control. He clutched his chest at the cold realization that he might be having a coronary. He felt dizzy and almost fell off the bar stool, but before he'd been able to cry for help—before anyone else in the bar had noticed him—the moment passed. Still dizzy, he managed to check his pulse; it was irregular and slightly fast.

The episode convinced him that he was not a well man. The next morning he telephoned my office for an appointment.

His final complaint, which Mr. Boyles had the insight and intelligence to present separately from his psychological and physical problems, was his decreased interest in sex. Now instead of leading his wife regularly into their private foreplay, he found himself pretending to be deeply involved in office work or inextricably absorbed in a basketball game on television. Actually he was afraid he could not finish what he started, a fear reinforced on several occasions by an inability to maintain his erection to climax. Though he had been careful to bring his wife to her own climax, neither had had their previous complete satisfaction.

"Dr. Parrish," he said sadly, "I don't even look at myself in the mirror when I shave." He sighed, and continued, "The wrinkles and the sags are bad enough, but lately it's my eyes I want to avoid; they're like a scared rabbit's."

I looked at him long and searchingly. While I would not want to accuse Ronald Boyles of exaggerating, if it were a rabbit he saw, it looked like one determined rabbit.

He was basically a positive man and I knew with the certainty of years of practice that he probably would have adjusted to his difficulties without my help. But he was not interested in simply learning to accept the changes in his person. He wanted more out of life than a passive acceptance. He was a man who enjoyed a good fight and now he was seeking me as his ally, which I was willing to be.

I gave him a most thorough physical examination. I checked his eyes for glaucoma and measured the vital capacity of his lungs. I examined his prostate fluid and took an electrocardiogram under stress. I palpated his abdomen, searched for enlarged lymph nodes, tested his reflexes, and with a sigmoidoscope scanned his colon for irregularities of the mucosal lining. I also tested his blood, urine, and feces, and had his sputum tested for malignant cells. I arranged to have him X-rayed from his elbow to his gallbladder, and several days later we had a conference to discuss the results.

Across the desk he looked like a man stoically expecting the worst. I had found nothing seriously wrong, but I knew that simply telling him this would not give him the reassurance he needed.

"Mr. Boyles, you had what I consider a complete examination. I know it has not been a pleasant experience, but I think it has been a profitable one. Using the most severe criteria, I have not discovered any significant abnormality. There is no evidence that you have any disease, or even any tendency to a serious pathological process."

It did not take a trained observer to see the muscles in his face relax in counterpoint to the straightening of his shoulders.

"However, the tests and my evaluation have uncovered a few abnormalities and enough nonspecific changes for me to conclude that your problem is the climacteric— the change of life."

"But Doctor," he said, somewhat taken aback, "I thought that was strictly a female complaint."

"The menopause is," I told him, "and people so closely

associate what they call the 'change of life' with the menopause per se that they ignore the fact that everyone who goes through middle age changes. For example, women become sterile. Though their functioning seldom comes to such an obvious halt, the primary sex glands in the male, the testes, usually loose some of their vigor with the passage of time. This can result in physical and mental changes due to an insufficient manufacture of their hormone, testosterone, as well as sexual problems and sterility.

"But hormone imbalances are not nearly so common in the male as in the female. Because there is no specific symptom or sign, like the menopause, to label it, the male 'change' has enjoyed more cocktail party commentary than serious medical attention. Doctors hesitate to make the diagnosis and patients do not like to accept it."

"Then what led you to conclude that my problem is the change of life?" he asked. "Have I given you any indication or have you found any evidence that makes you think I have a hormonal imbalance?"

"No. But the climacteric, especially in the male, can revolve around a core of mental and physical phenomena other than weak sex glands.

"In the first place, your fear of heart trouble brought you to consult me. Then after speaking with you and examining you, a variety of factors led me to my diagnosis, not the least of which was the absence of any definite pathological process. It is the general picture I see: several borderline abnormalities and nonspecific dysfunctions combined with and colored by your recent emotional stress.

"I can find nothing wrong with your heart. What you experienced at your club was a transient cardiac irregularity. These moments, sometimes only seconds, when your heart loses its normal rhythm are fairly common. Without any evidence of cardiac disease they mean little or nothing. The irregularity is a mixture of ineffectively weak contractions and compensatory strong, rapid ones. Sometimes the blood is not circulated properly, and if the brain suffers a fleeting lack of oxygen, you feel faint.

"Such episodes of light-headedness, skipped beats, and palpitations can be caused by a variety of factors, such as emotional upheavals, or unrelated physical disorders. During the male climacteric, palpitations are often associated with periods of crisis.

"Remember how frequently my nurses checked your blood pressure and counted your pulse? They noted only one irregularity in the beat, but the readings of your pressure varied widely, several slightly high. I looked hard for some specific physical abnormality, but I am happy to say, I found none. So I came to the conclusion, just as I did about your palpitations, that these transient disruptions in the expected behavior of your circulatory system had nothing to do with its basic health. It was doing nothing more than noting the stress and instability that you are experiencing. Many aspects of your life are changing and they are demanding your attention.

"Consider your symptoms: fatigue, insomnia, irritability, indecision, headaches, and complaints from your digestive and urinary tracts. All of these are so susceptible to such a variety of physical and psychological influences that it is difficult to say what exactly is the primary cause.

"Your urinary frequency and urgency is an example. This could have been due to a slight enlargement of your prostate, which is not uncommon in men your age. But your prostate is normal in size. And the X-rays of your stomach did not show any abnormality that could explain your acid indigestion. So for now, I feel safe to assume that both are a result of your anxiety.

"One of your liver function tests was elevated, but I

suspected it was just a laboratory error, which happens in screening profiles, so I repeated it by a more accurate procedure. The result was normal. But I had to consider your history of an increased consumption of alcohol. Using it to pacify your depression could have resulted in aggravating your liver. But, at the same time, I can be reasonably sure that the drinking problem is a direct result of your anxiety and depression."

"You're right there, Doctor," he agreed, though glumly.

"And you have given me some good reasons why you would be emotionally distraught. Fortunately, none of them poses any immediate threat, but some require attention. You realized that you had to get your physical and mental health in order before you could properly cope."

"Right again."

"I think I can provide the help you need," I said. "One last thing. Because you presented it to me separately, I want to discuss it separately: your loss of interest in sex. I think you may be underestimating the part this played in your dilemma. An active and satisfying sex life has been an integral factor in what has been, on the whole, a good life. Now that this part of life has turned sour, your sexual difficulties can only have exacerbated your other problems.

"Again, I'm happy to say that there is nothing physically wrong. Your tests indicate no hormone deficiency of any sort and there is no prostate or related difficulties that could be a contributing factor. As I said before, it is difficult during the climacteric to pair up every symptom with a specific cause. But I believe that your minor sexual difficulties are the result of nothing more than your anxiety over those same difficulties. We will keep in close touch over the next few months, monitoring the change you are going through. And I can assure you that your sexual problem is going to take care of itself."

"That's good news Dr. Parrish," he said. "It takes a lot of pressure off my mind, although I must admit, I'm not too happy with your diagnosis of the male menopause."

"Wait," I told him, "that's not my diagnosis. I said male climacteric. A man has no menopause. What's more, 'climacteric' is, as far as I'm concerned, appropriately positive. It comes from the Greek, meaning 'rung of a ladder.' It is a phase of life, a rung on the ladder, just like puberty. But it can give us a new perspective. As a result of this perspective, or any new perspective, in fact, we may find we have to alter our life in some way. Therein lies the second problem, and meaning, of climacteric, also from the Greek—crisis. The problems of adjustment can cause a crisis. It may not be pleasant, but it may be necessary. In coping with the crisis it is up to us to solve those problems so that whatever way we direct our lives from that point, the rungs we climb afterward will definitely be steps upward."

I noticed Mr. Boyles glancing at his watch. Two weeks before he had been reluctant to leave. Today, he seemed anxious to be on his way. I thought that was a good sign, so I quickly outlined my schedule of therapy. I gave him a prescription for a psychic energizer that also had a mild tranquilizing effect. In addition, he would get an injection of vitamins every week.

For the first two months I saw Mr. Boyles for counseling on weekly visits. During this time a change, almost a return to his former self, was obvious. He was gradually resuming a more active sex life and was trying hard to get his life in order. But he still had problems in the office. He was obviously pushing himself close to the edge of his endurance. I considered advising him to take a vacation, but experience had taught me that even if he had agreed, the vacation would have little therapeutic value. Intense and conscientious men cannot relax when they know that their return means only a resumption of even more problems than they left behind.

Thus, I was surprised when four months later Ronald Boyles came in to discuss stopping the psychic energizer. He was off on a vacation and did not feel he would need it.

"I'm glad you've decided to take some time off," I told him. "You must feel you have your life pulled back into shape."

"Not altogether," he admitted, "but for the time at least I have things under control, and I certainly could use the rest. I must admit, though, I've got another reason up my sleeve. . . ."

"Yes?"

"There's a board meeting at my firm next week to select a new executive vice-president. I figured the members would be impressed that one of the candidates felt sufficiently secure not to hang around to remind them of his qualifications. So, I'm taking the family down to Mexico. I'll be back to see you in three weeks."

He came back to a promotion as well.

The climacteric, though it may be difficult to identify, is as much a period of life as childhood or old age. It is an integral part of the progressive pattern of development, fruition, decline, and rest that constitute the life cycle.

The factor common to all these phases is change, and in the climacteric this change is frequently dramatic. For all who live past forty, male and female alike, change is inevitable. The fifth and sixth decades are the years when we reap the benefits of our efforts, assess our position in life, and make realistic plans for the future. They are busy years, full years, but different years. Altering our patterns of thinking and of living during the climacteric is necessary to prepare us for the years to come. Some of the changes are stimulating, others are depressing, many are bittersweet. The excitement of vague dreams is replaced by the comfort of practical plans. The gambling on outside chances—so attractive in youth when years lie ahead in which to recover from possible failure—is exchanged for stability.

Just as adolescence is a hectic era of growing up, the climacteric is preoccupied with the problems of growing older. The necessary professional, social, and familial adjustments of the climacteric are made even more critical by biological developments. What form the climacteric takes is an individual matter, with a definite gender difference. But both men and women go through similar evolutions in their personal, professional, and social lives, and both are subjected to degenerative physical changes.

Whatever form it takes, the climacteric is always there. No doubt one of the reasons there has been so little serious attempt to define and recognize it is that we passively accept these changes as natural and inevitable. While they are, to some extent, they do not have to be as severe or as unexpected as they often are. We know what to do and we know what to look for and we should do both.

The early manifestations of the male climacteric are gradual. Time may creep up on us slowly, but creep it does. Without noticing it, a man in his forties may find himself holding his evening newspaper an inch or two farther away for easier reading. Or maybe his favorite reading lamp suddenly requires a brighter bulb. And the whites of his eyes, for no apparent reason, appear red. He needs glasses. For those men whose vision has always been normal, learning to keep a pair of glasses at hand is an adjustment—perhaps the first of the climacteric.

Meanwhile, other problems crop up. His teeth, after several decades of unprotesting service, can now sentence him to long hours in the dentist's chair. Gray hair appears, and worse still, there are signs of baldness. At the same time there is increased hair growth on other parts of the body; bristles sprout inside the nose and in the ears.

The skin becomes dry and looses its elasticity. The skin texture becomes rough in some spots and thin in others. Acnelike eruptions and blotches may add to its irregular appearance. Frequently, there are changes in body contour, due to excess fat.

Overweight is not exclusively a curse of middle age. But the distortions that fat deposits make in middle age are more obvious because of the loss in muscle tone that accompanies aging. Pot bellies protrude over the belt. Big thighs are not just fat but are now covered with small tiers of skin that has wrinkled because it has lost its tone and the support of underlying musculature and connective tissue. These changes do not have to be as marked as they frequently are. But by avoiding exercise and rationalizing an increasingly sedentary life, we passively encourage them.

Inactivity fosters another typical problem of middle age: rheumatism, a nonspecific inflammatory disease of the connective tissues, including bone and ligaments. Though rarely used today as a diagnosis by physicians, it immediately paints in the mind of the layman the picture of sore and stiff joints and muscles. When it attacks the joints, usually the large ones, it is called rheumatoid arthritis. For no obvious reason a knee temporarily becomes red, hot, swollen, and tender. Since it tends to migrate, an elbow or a shoulder aches, especially when it has been the site of a previous injury, or, as anyone's grandmother would quickly agree, the weather is changing for the worse.

The rims of the spinal vertebrae, especially in the neck, can deteriorate to the point where a simple turn of the head triggers a shock of pain. Muscles alone can become achy and sore, as if they had a cold in them. And not infrequently isolated areas of numbness in the skin, which is usually attributed to "poor circulation," is a sign of rheumatism. No one knows exactly what causes this degenerative change in the musculoskeletal system, but it is obvious that disuse aggravates the condition. After even a short period of inactivity an afflicted area develops soreness and stiffness that improve with mobility.

Even without the complication of rheumatism, one's body language is not as glib as it once was. A middle-aged man walks neither as fast nor with the spring he was accustomed to. With muscle and connective tissue deteriorating, rather than revitalizing, there is a decrease in strength and elasticity. Without these to sustain and coordinate finer movements, he loses some of his grace and agility.

He avoids walking up hills because he lacks the strength and he does not dance every dance because he lacks endurance. If he should manage to dance the night away, he is acutely aware of his effort the next morning. He is out of shape. These limitations are not inevitable, but they can be predicted with certainty in a man who avoids physical activity. Just because he is older, and is no doubt busy and pressed for time, does not mean that he should confine his movements only to those that are necessary. His body suffers the consequences of his laziness. His mind is quite content that he spends an entire afternoon lying on the beach. But when he gets ready to go home, his muscles will complain that they have not been challenged even by an easy Australian crawl.

In the climacteric, a man's body knows, if he doesn't, that there is a special meaning to the old saying that he is not as young as he used to be. It is only natural that with usage and time changes occur in his body. And these are by no means limited to those that can be seen. Internally his organs do not operate as efficiently as they did once. He does not seem to recover from a disease or injury with his accustomed speed. Basic physiologic processes, such as oxygen exchange in the lungs and tissues and the assimilation and elimination of food, tend to be more sluggish and ineffective. Having to cater to basic functions previously taken for granted is a bore. And boring, too, are his easy fatigability, temporary and minor disorders in organs as disparate as his tear ducts and his bladder, and symptoms he had disdained in others, such as back trouble and headaches. Then there are symptoms such as chest pains and coughs that are more a worry than a bore.

The back trouble is probably due to poor posture, the headache to tension, the chest pain to a sore muscle between the ribs, and the cough to irritated bronchi. But each symptom could have a more important meaning. Thus, to note them isn't sufficient if we then do nothing about them. Still better, is to detect them before they become a problem. The only way to do that is to consult a physician and request a thorough examination. We are much less likely to need his treatment if we do not neglect or insult our body, which unfortunately cannot continue to offer us the efficient services we demand.

Rather than worry and complain, it is better to take a manly step and see a doctor. After putting test results together with a complete medical history, he can assure his patient about the absence (or treatment, should it be necessary) of degenerative diseases. What are degenerative diseases? Everything from hypertension, anemia, glaucoma, hernia, prostatitis, and high blood fats, to arthritis, arteriosclerosis, diabetes, emphysema, cancer, and an enlarged heart. That is a lot of reassurance!

Why then, don't more men consult a doctor before illness strikes? Maybe the man doesn't want to be compromised by admitting his weaknesses or assuming the embarrassing positions and being subjected to impersonal poking and bloodletting necessary for a thorough physical. Or maybe he simply doesn't want to part with the money or the time. More than likely he is afraid of what the doctor might tell him. So, like Carl Rivensen, he delays until confronted with a problem he just cannot ignore.

Carl Rivensen described himself as a simple man. He was also quiet and serious, an attitude exaggerated by his present depression. He was sixty-one, and an accountant with a large insurance firm. He lived with his wife and children in a home they owned, and his life had settled into an easy and satisfying routine. On Tuesday evening he bowled, on Saturday he attended to chores, on Sunday morning he ushered at church, and twice a week he and his wife played cards with friends. Other evenings he worked on his collection of picture postcards or hand-tooled leather belts, which he gave away. He did not want to retire, but he was ready if the company insisted. But for the last two years he had found this routine increasingly tiring. He had frequently begged off from his obligations and neglected his hobbies. He said he had no energy or enthusiasm. Getting up in the morning was a chore. The ride to work exhausted him. On the job he did only the things he had to and then mechanically. As soon as he came home he ate then sat and stared into space waiting to go to bed. He felt his life was, in his words, "slipping away."

At times, for no reason at all, he would start crying. No, he hadn't anything particularly sad on his mind. Maybe he would think about his family and feel guilty that he had not done more for them. Still, he believed his wife when she told him that if the next three generations uplifted the family as much as he had, his great grandchildren would be senators and millionaires.

He offered no further symptom, but on questioning I learned that his sleep was poor and that his appetite, usually good, was now off. He also had to urinate frequently, getting up two or three times a night, then experiencing difficulty urinating. He sometimes felt a tingling sensation in his fingers.

His physical examination was normal except that his knee jerk and ankle reflexes were moderately reduced and his prostate gland was definitely enlarged and soft. When I told him this, I saw a glint in his eyes. After I added that I also had found pus and cellular debris in his prostate fluid, he relaxed a little and asked if that gland had something to do with reproduction and sex. When I told him it did, he said, "maybe that is the cause of it all."

He went on to explain that until now he had not known how to bring up the subject that worried him most. It was impossible for him to get an erection. The difficulty had been developing for several years, but for the last three months he had not had an erection or an ejaculation. Admittedly he had been tired and blue before then, but with this latest problem his anxiety and depression had overwhelmed him.

"My wife and I have always enjoyed each other's company. I think our closeness in bed kept us a happy family. I know that it saw us through many an emergency, and made us content when we had a lot of reasons to be miserable. Until this problem started we had relations at least two or three times a week. I still want to; but I just cannot do it. All of the feelings are there, but nothing happens. We've tried everything, including some of the things in those books. Of course, she tries to pretend nothing is seriously wrong, just a phase all men my age go through. She even says it's her fault. But I'm afraid she thinks I've lost interest in her and I haven't. I never could. Something has to be wrong with my body. I guess you found it, the prostate."

Mr. Rivensen's assumption had some merit. Diseases of the prostate can impair sexual functioning, and his was both infected and enlarged. Prostatitis, infection or inflammation, occurs in all age groups. Enlargement, benign hypertrophy as opposed to malignant growth, is common in older men, appearing in roughly half the male population over sixty, though it may begin in even younger men. But I doubted that either of these was the primary cause of his total impotency. Other factors, psychological or physical, had to be involved. No doubt his emotional state was implicated, and I was becoming more convinced there was also a hormone factor.

In males, there is a syndrome of endocrine imbalance similar to the menopausal syndrome in women. The "Leydig cells" of the testes stop secreting the amount of testosterone the body needs. Through the same type of feedback mechanism that operates between it and the ovaries, the pituitary gland responds to the deficiency of testosterone by sending out more hormone messengers to stimulate the testes. The results of this change in hormone balance are not unlike hot flashes and sweats produced in women.

On a hunch, I asked Mr. Rivensen if he'd ever experienced any such symptoms. He thought for a moment. "I don't know, Doctor. Nothing lately that I can remember. But a couple of years ago, I recall a few times when my skin seemed to tingle and feel feverish. I tried not to pay it attention and sometimes it would be over in a few minutes. Other times it lasted so long I felt suffocated. I would have to loosen my tie and take my jacket off. Then I would sweat considerably. But it would pass, and I didn't bother about it. Altogether, it only lasted a few months."

I remember how his muscles seemed exceptionally flabby, his testicles small and rubbery, and his hair distribution sparse; all symptoms of testosterone deficiency. I was convinced we should investigate this possibility further, even though a primary testosterone deficiency alone is rare. In hardly more than 10 percent of the cases of impotency, is testosterone deficiency the sole etiology.

Relative deficiencies may be implicated in other cases. By increasing a patient's testosterone level with medication, I have had some success in restoring expected potency. Occasionally, I will give hormone injections in cases where I know the impotence is purely psychological and any improvement likely to be the result of a placebo effect. That is, because a man believes the injection will work, it produces the desired response. The important thing is to make the man feel something is being done to help him. And even in the absence of a demonstrable deficiency, there is evidence of a positive biochemical effect that the male hormone has on the brain. Possibly only a slight increase in active testosterone can change a man's negative outlook on life to a positive one. Had I not been so certain of Ronald Boyles' ability to pull himself through his difficulties with a minimum of treatment, I might have considered such injections in his case.

Carl Rivensen was a different situation altogether. After recommending hot baths and prescribing an antibiotic for his prostatitis, I told him to collect a twenty-four hour specimen of urine to be analyzed for hormones. I would see him in a week to review the results of his tests.

At that time I told him he was right in thinking there was a physical basis for his major complaints, fatigue and impotence. Both his blood and his urine showed that his testicles were not functioning properly. The amount of male hormone they were secreting was only 25 percent of normal and the depressed hormone levels weakened his muscle tissue and possibly adversely affected the biochemistry of his brain. The fatigue also had been aggravated by his depression. But that factor, too, would be alleviated once he was started on supplemental testosterone. The hormone would most likely reinstate his potency, which would, in turn, have a dramatic effect on his sense of well-being.

"You are a lucky man, Mr. Rivensen. I'll tell you now that when you consulted me, my initial impression was that your problems were fundamentally psychological. Both depression and impotency are frequent complaints at your age, but in spite of a vested interest, physicians have not found a quick and reliable remedy for either or both. But your case is an exception. It has a simple cause, a primary hormone deficiency that can be easily treated. All that has to be done is to supply you with the testosterone you cannot manufacture yourself. But don't expect a miracle. It will take a little time for the therapy to work. Furthermore, since you haven't been able to have an ejaculation and clean out your prostate, the congestion and inflammation, even some of the enlargement, will take a while to subside. You will have to be patient, but only for a few months. Then I think you will be agreeably surprised by the results."

Though physical complaints multiply as we grow older, psychiatric disorders are frequently the underlying reason men consult a doctor during the middle years. The male climacteric is characterized more by emotional than by physical disease. But the doctor must be astute enough to gently probe the superficial symptoms to discover the real cause for the patient's visit.

The average middle-aged man is naturally anxious about the future of his personal and professional life. Important decisions face him at the same time that he is becoming more aware of his physical mortality.

He is concerned with establishing his professional stability, and afraid of lowering his sights and settling for less than his early ambitions. One of his agonies may be guilt that he has not been more successful. He may be disillusioned by the cold, selfish manipulations of his business world, as well as by a growing awareness of the absence of kindness and consideration in his daily intercourse with other humans. He is resentful that a manager who has been with the company only six years has been promoted to a department head. Or he is just as disturbed by the dismissal of a clerk who has been there longer than he. He is angry at the injustices of life, which seem to reward qualities he doesn't have or understand, while ignoring competency and dedication, which he is willing and able to give. No wonder he is nervous, indecisive. He does not know where he stands. He does not know what to do.

Not only is he frustrated, he is restless. He might like a change, but is afraid to make one. Perhaps he actually looked for a new job, as a support to his faltering ego, and was offered one. It may have seemed more interesting and had a better title, but not much more money. Should he take the risk now, with the children in school and the market so low that he'd get little from his profit-sharing plan? No, there is too much at stake. He might be willing to risk it if he looked younger. He knows how much appearances count today; a spry step, a full head of hair with no gray, and a smooth, unlined face. He understands now why the market for male cosmetics is booming. He resolves to stop eating so much and to get more sleep. He will exercise, too, if only he can find some time. He knows that pulling himself together would be a way to start putting his life together. Maybe the girls would start looking at him again. And the first time one does, he tells himself, he is going to return the compliment.

So he decides he needs a love affair. But what if he gets caught? Divorce, distress, frozen food, loneliness, disapproval from friends and his employer. Still it would be rejuvenating to know some attractive woman desired him. It might not be all that dangerous and possibly it would be one way to cope with all the changes he feels. He might not have to leave his wife. All he wants is a change of pace, a little happiness for a little while.

But happiness seems to elude him. Some measure of depression is always with him. No matter what aspect of his life he considers, changes and adjustments have to be made. Yet his powers of concentration, so necessary for decision, seem poor. Random thoughts, even when reading or watching a movie, repeatedly distract him. Where did all these worries come from? He had problems when he was young, but they did not seem so threatening, so real.

Often what men want most to escape is the realization that age is creeping up. Many men still cling to outdated conceptions of gender roles; for example, the male should always be strong physically and mentally and avoid showing weakness at all cost. Not infrequently that cost can be very high.

Men, like women, often try to stop the clock. In the way they dress and groom themselves, they attempt to look younger than their years. In their activities, too, they try to prove they are full of the vigor of budding potential. Carried to extremes, that reaction can be inappropriate, sometimes pathetically so, leading to a kind of frantic overcompensation that not infrequently accompanies the male climacteric. Dayton Killibrew was a prime example of such manic behavior.

Ten minutes late for his appointment, Dayton Killibrew dashed by the nurse into the examining room and apologizing profusely thanked me repeatedly for seeing him on a "matter of utmost urgency."

He was late because his job interview had lasted longer than he had expected. He had been laid off when the advertising company he worked for had had to make some cutbacks in personnel, and had given him three months to find a new position. He was not worried, however. As a rare commodity in today's job market, he wanted a position that would "appreciate and reward his creativity and productivity." If he could not find that, he was ready to start his own business, even if he had to use his savings and put a second mortgage on his home.

I looked at him. He was well into his forties, not fat, but a little overweight. His suit was expensively tailored, but the long flared jacket and the bell-bottomed pants were too tight. His shirt, a bright green, was also too severely cut; as he moved, the skin of his stomach bulged through the gaps between the buttons. As he reached into his pocket for a cigarette, bracelets jangled and he continued to give me a history I had not asked for. Yet, it turned out to be relevant.

He continued his rapid monologue, explaining that in his business, advertising, it was necessary to be "in there swinging with the times, actually a little ahead of them and with a flare." He was living and loving like every day was a honeymoon. It was expensive, but the impression he was creating was worth the money. Finally, coming around to his reason for seeking my services, the loving had had an unexpected side effect. Recently he had noticed a cluster of tiny scabs on his penis.

"How long have they been there?" I asked.

"About six or seven days. I wanted to come earlier, but I couldn't find the time. They started as small blisters."

I examined him. "I think I can almost assure you it isn't a syphilis chancre. However, I'm going to take a blood test."

"I was worried about gonorrhea."

"Its symptoms are completely different, a discharge from the penis. This is typical of herpes."

"Herpes, you mean like a cold sore? I have them frequently on my lip. How did I get them down there?"

"In the last ten years it has become a very common veneral disease," I explained, at the same time assuring him it could be treated.

"What about my wife?" he asked, tucking his shirt in his pants, lighting another cigarette, and looking at his watch.

"When did you last have intercourse?"

"With her? That was over a month ago."

"Has she had any signs or symptoms?"

"She hasn't mentioned them. But then since I got fired—positioned off I mean—we've sort of drifted apart."

"Then probably she has not been infected. But I advise you to avoid contact with anyone until we get the results of your blood test."

"But I've got a date tonight after the job interview."

"Why not cancel it?"

He seemed somewhat relieved. "If those are your orders, Doctor."

Before he left the examining room I suggested that he

have his blood pressure checked. I was not surprised to see that it was elevated, and I told him I suspected he needed treatment for hypertension. He should make an appointment for a more complete examination when he returned for his blood test result. He barely acknowledged my suggestion with a quick nod before rushing out the door and on to his next appointment.

The primary difference between Dayton Killibrew and men like Ronald Boyles or Carl Rivensen is that Dayton was in trouble and did not know it. Instead of facing the problems of middle life, he was running from them.

Carl Rivensen would have been amazed, even envious of Dayton's sex life. If a man has a sexual problem in the climacteric more frequently it is a decrease in sex drive and performance. It is important to point out that barring a testosterone deficiency, impotency is often an expression of an eroded ego. The stress and insecurity of change threatens the sense of masculinity. Dayton Killibrew, under the protection of an overcompensating psyche, was able to bolster his stunned ego with the sexual gratification he got from extramarital relationships. However, this defensive maneuver prevented him from coming to grips with the reality of his situation.

Dayton was a personality medical science refers to as "Type A." People with this behavior are always rushing against time. Even if their lives naturally necessitate hectic schedules, they manage to increase the pressure. Everyone knows the type: by trying to do the "something extra," they frequently end up accomplishing less than they would have if they had not overextended themselves. They are highly competitive, anxious to win, and frustrated by losing. Rest and relaxation is foreign to their nature. They work crossword puzzles while they watch television. Their outward mannerisms and attitudes are frenetic; inwardly they are tense and irritable. Patience is not one of their virtues. They feel that life is passing them by and are forever frantically trying to fill every second of it.

Dayton was a super "Type A." In view of his agitated state, I was surprised that he kept his next appointment at all. He was late, of course, and before I started to examine him he informed me that he had an important interview in half an hour. I noticed that when he undressed for the examination he did not remove his watch. Furthermore, on the watchband he had clipped a metal calendar of the month. He was pressured not only by the hour, but by the days and the weeks.

My examination revealed he was a primary cardiac risk. He smoked two to three packages of cigarettes a day; he was twenty-one pounds overweight; his blood pressure was high; his father had died at age fifty-eight of a heart attack; and his mother had diabetes and arteriosclerosis. The abnormal amount of lipids in his blood (cholesterol and triglycerides) and his electrocardiogram, which suggested coronary insufficiency, made it clear: if he did not take care, he was likely to have a heart attack.

I had to level with him. As I told him of his condition, I saw an ego disintegrate. He confided that he had failed to find a new job, and had exhausted his prospects. He had given up the notion of starting a business of his own. He and his wife were hardly civil to one another; he still had a son to put through college; and his house was not only mortgaged, but in need of repair. His savings, what was left after his recent fling, would carry his family for perhaps six months. He now realized that every month counted in getting employment.

I had no doubt Mr. Killibrew was bright and probably talented. But though he was still trying to put up a good front, there was a note of desperation beneath his bravado. He was not just at a crossroad—he was in limbo. He was in need of direction.

"The first thing you have to do," I told him, "for the sake of your family as well as for yourself, is to let your body know you do not intend to be the victim of its changes. I will prescribe medication to lower your cholesterol and your blood pressure. But pills can't do it all. I am putting you on a special diet, and you must also make an effort to get more exercise. Your body is suffering from years of neglect."

My patient was hardly alone in his neglect of himself. He ate what he liked and avoided exercise. Such lassitude has become a way of life for most of today's men. Their excuse is usually their work, which occupies so much of their time or tires them so that they limit their activity to necessary movements. Living by his brain, modern man has forgotten he was a creature of nature long before he began to think. To improve his general health and attractiveness, the climacteric male should adopt some regular schedules and habits as to exercise, sleep, and proper diet.

He should also dress carefully and appropriately. He should be proud of his age and of how well his age can look. This pride should carry over into everything he does. Erect posture, expanding the chest and contracting the abdominal muscles, can create a more genuinely impressive appearance than any expensive suit, and also guard against back trouble. He should remember that people think of him as he thinks of himself and the most important element of a commanding appearance is an inner security.

"You must also get yourself into a better frame of mind," I continued. "I will prescribe something for that also. This particular medication will relieve your anxiety and most likely elevate your mood enough to let some constructive thoughts break through that circle of worry. You can also use them for sleep."

I was pleased to see Mr. Killibrew look at me directly. "I was going to ask you for sleeping pills, but I was afraid to." He slowly and deliberately lit a cigarette, a habit smokers practice when giving serious consideration to a matter.

"I'm not going to tell you to stop smoking right now. While you're getting your life into focus, you'll need some crutches. But, you understand that in the not too distant future you will have to find a less destructive pacifier."

"You make it all sound so easy Doctor; it's not. Particularly since I'm afraid I've lost my most valuable support, my wife. She's stood by me, put my head together, and pulled me through a thousand difficulties before. Oh, she's no angel, but she can always put her finger right on the nut of a problem. She is also a fighter. She has been going through the change of life, but instead of its throwing her, it seems to have given her strength; too much I'm afraid. She is talking about getting a job herself; or a divorce. I know I can't fight this without her help."

Dayton Killibrew was not unique in his dependency on his wife at this time of life. During the trauma of the climacteric, a wife can offer the kind of support that no friend, physician, or psychiatrist can. She can offer him the feeling that whatever the problem, it is not just his, it is theirs. They can fight it together and they can survive it together.

In the climacteric a man tends to become insecure and indecisive. Preoccupied with his failures rather than his successes, he is frightened. This fear can express itself in the numbing depression of Carl Rivensen, or in the frenetic anxiety of Dayton Killibrew. The portent of change, real or imagined, becomes a serious threat to the man's existing life situation, however unhappy the present might be. He simply does not feel strong enough to cope. In his search for strength, the first person he usually turns to is his wife.

I was afraid Mr. Killibrew's wife might be the type to pull the foundation out from under her husband's tottering ego. With unrelenting criticism and repeated I-told-you-sos she could easily scuttle any progress he made in reorganizing the scattered forces of his life. I thought it might be a good idea to talk with her, and suggested that she accompany Dayton on his next visit—ostensibly to discuss his diet.

Mary Killibrew was not at all what I expected. She would not have impressed anyone with her brilliance or chic and she did not care. Perhaps because she had faced the facts of her own climacteric change, she had recognized her husband's problem long before he had. Her threats of striking out on her own had been aimed at shocking him back into reality. She had been quietly pruning their life-style to prepare for the financial limitations she anticipated.

As basic as she was practical, she made no attempt to hide her anger at his recent adventures and extravagances.

"Doctor Parrish," she said, when her husband had gone into the next room to have his blood pressure taken, "I don't mind telling you that it's not easy to live with Dayton. But then I've never fooled myself into thinking that marriage was an easy proposition. I've worked hard, and so has he, to make our marriage work, and I'm not going to quit now."

With determination such as that, it was not difficult to impress on her the importance of encouraging her husband to take care of himself. I also suspected she would be a strong support in helping him regain his shattered sense of security and self-confidence.

Dayton Killibrew ultimately found his security in a new setting and a new life-style. He got a job in a small city. The pay was less, but so were his living expenses. The money he got from the sale of his Connecticut home paid for one that he liked more and was only ten minutes from his new job. And the bank owned only a small share of it. In his work he was not going to create national slogans, but he no longer felt a need to. He was secure. He may have lost the battle of Madison Avenue, but he had won the war of his climacteric.

What was for Dayton Killibrew a realistic compromise would for others be an unnecessary sacrifice. The climacteric by no means always requires a modification of ambition, a "settling for less." Rather it requires, even demands, some realistic evaluation and some practical decisions. Facing the climacteric may neither guarantee a promotion like Ronald Boyles' nor necessitate an accommodation like Dayton Killibrew's, but it will assure a happier life, and a fuller one.

The Crisis in the Mirror

Cosmetics and Skin Care

———

The crisis in the mirror—the moment a woman sees herself as an individual who is getting older—can be traumatic. Often, this response is treated as an exaggeration or overreaction, and the woman who experiences fear or sadness at the recognition of new lines, wrinkles, or other changes in her appearance is thought of as shallow, selfish, and vain.

Such reactions to the aging process are not expressions of mere vanity. Instead, sadness, fear, and even tears are legitimate by-products of a society that worships youth and turns the later years of life into a lonely and often tragic experience.

"Youth culture" has become a life-style as well as a catch phrase for what amounts to a national obsession. Youth and beauty are seen as synonymous; therefore age and ugliness have become equated. The woman who notices that her skin seems dulled and drooping and finds herself crying isn't shedding tears for what has gone, at least not exclusively. Memories may, in fact, be a comfort.

78

She may be far more upset, and rightly so, by the unknown future. She senses that she has come to a turning point in life, and the signpost's message seems to be written in the newly discovered lines and wrinkles she contemplates. Old age is coming closer, or she is moving toward it. She considers, perhaps for the first time, a change in her point of identification. Time itself, coupled with dysfunctions of her body that she cannot fully comprehend, seems to be leading her to a role which too frequently lies outside the mainstream of society.

Just how a woman reacts, of course, is a matter of attitude, environment, and general sense of well-being. One who is secure in her family and other intimate relationships may face the mirror comfortably. The woman who is generally unfulfilled, or who relies heavily on her physical appearance in relating to the world, may have a more serious problem. The woman who has already experienced other symptoms of the change of life may have been prepared by her physician, and acceptance may be easier.

For many women, however, the change in their appearance is the first sign of the climacteric. Before degenerative changes in other organs, including the ovaries, manifest themselves, a visible physical change may bring them to the doctor's office.

There may be no more medical help needed than some psychological support, some advice on skin and hair care, and in some cases the prescription of special skin creams. Growing older, however, is a continual process. Other changes, not all of them so visible as lines and wrinkles, are certain to follow. It is an excellent opportunity for a physician to involve his patient in a positive regimen for preventing, where possible, and treating the other phenomena of aging. I recall the history of one such patient, who had come to me after a particularly painful confrontation with the mirror.

Janet Milam had been late leaving the office and Arthur was due in half an hour. She pulled off her earrings, put them on top of the dresser, and had just unclasped her beads when she looked into the mirror. Startled, she took a step backward and cocked her head to the side.

She was seeing a middle-aged woman. Coming closer, she scrutinized from all angles the image that followed in syncopation her slightly frantic movements. There was no doubt: the middle-aged woman was herself.

What had happened?

She'd had a good night's sleep, and with a two-hour luncheon, her day could hardly have been called a rough one. She wasn't sick and had not been bothered by any of those fleeting flushes she had had the month before. In fact, she felt better than she had for a week. Nor was she worried about anything. Her father back home in South Carolina was recovering nicely from a bout with pneumonia, and Arthur was as attentive as ever. Even her own emotional anxiety over Arthur—where was it leading and when—had begun to seem silly. She had caught herself daydreaming about him several times during the day and had planned his favorite meal for dinner.

Yet she looked ten years older than she had that morning. The pattern of lines and creases she had noticed on middle-aged women at the office was now right there in the mirror, on her own face. She cut her eyes sideways to inspect her profile. The little lumps below the corners of her mouth were no longer visible, but the bags under her eyes were, if anything, more prominent, and she thought she detected a double chin. Slowly turning to consult herself full-face again, she threw her head back and stretched her neck. She looked down her nose into the mirror and was relieved to find that the extra chin had disappeared. But the relief was momentary. She remembered having read about an aging actress who always insisted on playing the role of a haughty woman. That might work for a few hours a day on the stage, but how could she go around the rest of her life with her nose up in the air?

Again she stared into the mirror, this time squinting her eyes, trying to get the effect of dim lights. The result was relatively agreeable. She would put rheostats and pink bulbs throughout the apartment. But how would she go to the office? Dark glasses? Maybe. A dark and mysterious woman. But what about the insipient double chin? A veil? Unrealistic, she concluded—not to mention out of fashion—but she *could* throw away all her turtlenecks.

A sigh escaped from her sinking chest, and her hands moved upward. With her thumbs she tucked some loose skin behind each earlobe, and with her fingers she tightened the skin over her cheeks and at the corners of her eyes. The result was pleasant. Plastic surgery! But what would people say? And what about her hands, whose reflection now caught her attention?

The wrinkled, dry texture of their skin seemed to offer no resistance to the bulging veins. And were those brown marks freckles or liver spots? Was it possible to perform plastic surgery on hands? A woman on television had said that anyone who had had her face lifted should either wear gloves or keep her hands away from her face. How could she do that when she had a habit of resting her chin on her fist? She looked again, trying to be objective. The wrinkles, chins, and veins were definitely there, but for some strange reason she seemed to be seeing them in a magnifying glass instead of a mirror. They had probably been developing over a long period of time, but she had been too busy to notice. Had she really thought she could live all those years and not look her age? The idea brought a pause to her racing mind. She was forty-eight, but had always been youthful looking and had, in fact, been passing herself off as ten years younger, even to her close friends. So far, she had managed to get away with it, though some of her more skeptical acquaintances may have suspected she was a year or two older.

Sometimes, even in her most private moments, she forgot how old she really was. But now, as she scrutinized herself, she looked closer to her actual age than to the one she professed.

But why did all this seem to happen at once—so quickly? It wasn't like the frown wrinkles that had crept across her brow. Their slow progress had given her time to get used to them. But the changes she was shocked by today were much more serious. She didn't see how she could become accustomed to them; furthermore, she didn't want to. She wanted to do something constructive. But what?

She looked at her hair. The untinted roots were longer than she had realized, but she was encouraged to see that the majority were her own color, not gray. The first straggling grays had been "interesting," she thought, something she hadn't even minded talking about. When her beauty operator had suggested a tinting she had been indifferent, even amused. At her age? But the rinse to homogenize the different colors and give her hair a fuller look had become a regular part of her beauty parlor regimen.

Remembering that women, too, can go bald, she examined her scalp, pulling at a few hairs that, to her satisfaction, held firm. She could detect no thinning. Even that wouldn't be so bad; she could wear a wig.

Dry, wrinkled skin was another matter. Forget about trying to actually make it smooth and supple again, she thought; she would be happy just to be able to create the illusion. She recalled reading something about elaborate treatments "guaranteed" to restore lost youth. Could they have any basis in fact?

She used various moisturizers, but had never taken the time to get onto a regular skin care regime. Some of her friends at the office did, and she tried to remember how their skin looked. Betty Fisher flashed into her mind. She had an elaborate routine that took her an hour or more a day. She experimented with everything new on the market and swore each was better than the next. Betty definitely had good skin.

Janet knew she was exaggerating her changes, but even so they presented her with more problems than she cared to imagine. She cursed herself for having looked in the mirror in the first place.

But the act of looking in the mirror was not, of course, the origin of her crisis. It was what she saw there. If it hadn't been today, then tomorrow, next week, or next year, her psyche would eventually have introduced her to this new woman—a face bearing only a faint resemblance to the picture of herself she kept in the locket of her unconscious. Whether she was ready or not, the time had come for a change. And, in a few days, she would be seeking constructive help in that change.

The changes a woman notices in her skin are due to a number of factors—some of them peculiar to our time. Air pollution, even fifty years ago, wasn't a major problem. Today we recognize that environmental pollutants can and do cause a number of skin problems, ranging from allergies to an acceleration of the physical aging process.

If changing times have brought new problems, they have also brought new insights and solutions into how life-style affects physical aging. Exposure to sunlight, we now know, unless judiciously moderated, can cause early lines and wrinkles, and even skin cancers. Today we also recognize the effects of diet in terms of the physical signs of aging—and we know that poor eating habits can speed up their appearance. Smoking, too, may take its toll, depositing toxins in the cells and causing a fine web of "smokers" lines around the mouth.

None of these factors is a primary cause of aging, but singly and cumulatively they are catalysts, accelerating, aggravating, and hastening the aging process. In her search for a way to hold onto youth, a woman sometimes forgets that aging, after all, is normal. Instead of being encouraged to look the best she can at her age, she is urged to cover up, conceal, and obliterate what Madison Avenue has termed the "telltale" signs; signs that are, in fact, normal to a woman of her years. Pressured and frightened, she may embark on a search for some nonexistent secret of youth. So involved can she become in searching for a cosmetic miracle that she loses her perspective. Fear and urgency replace reason and judgment.

Cosmetics can be beneficial, enhancing not only the physical image but the sense of well-being. But in our effort to understand the skin, we must first forget the popular message of the cosmetic advertisements—"your skin was meant to look young"—and must reassess the purposes nature intended for it. In terms of the body, the skin is a container, outlining and protecting internal organs and systems. The largest organ of all, the skin is like a shield, protecting the body and its parts (most of which are far more delicate and far less capable of environmental defense) from a number of factors. Changes in climate and temperature, and even simple sunlight, could be deadly were it not for the moderating and protective capactities of the skin. It protects, in addition, against the invasion of microorganisms.

The skin also serves as an outward reflection of physical and mental well-being. When we are embarrassed, for example, the blood vessels in the skin dilate, producing a blush of color. When we are frightened, they constrict, giving the pallor of fear. An abundance of healthy red corpuscles gives the rosy glow of good health; anemic blood, lacking in iron, is seen in an ashen cast. Nervousness can reflect itself in the skin, and increasingly science is finding links between anxiety and a number of rashes, irritations, and other disorders of the skin. In the same way, changes in other organs of the body are reflected. Liver disorders, gallbladder problems, and diseases of the pancreas can cause jaundice, a yellowing of the skin. Often this can be one of the first signs of such diseases—the crucial signal that brings a patient to a doctor for essential treatment.

The skin also serves as an organ of excretion. We sweat all the time, though the rate of activity of the sweat glands is increased by temperature, exercise, and anxiety. Excessive sweating, in severe or prolonged cases, can gravely endanger the fluid balance of the body. Normal sweating, however, is a life-assuring function through which the body eliminates a solution of sodium chloride and other substances.

These are but a few of the things that the skin does, or aids in. Books can and have been written on that subject alone, and new discoveries are helping science to add new chapters. One thing, however, is apparent. Nature has designed the skin to play a key role in general health and well-being. Looking beautiful, as far as nature is concerned, is purely coincidental!

Yet it is natural for us to want to look our best, and best can mean better than nature intended. Degenerative change, in even the most healthy individual, is natural; a woman of forty simply cannot look twenty, as much as she might like to. None of us has found the fabled fountain of youth, nor has science, despite important breakthroughs, unlocked the mystery of why we age.

We do, however, know that as we age, changes take place. Many of these changes directly affect the way we look—and make us look older. The body, like a computer, is programmed. To a large extent, the aging process is "built in" to our basic makeup.

How we live can accelerate the process of aging, as we have discussed, but the rules are not hard and fast. The general recommendations made by science—against smoking, excessive exposure to sun, etc.—are based on general observation. Yet it must be said that there are those individuals who can and do break all the rules, making all the mistakes without showing any apparent ill effect. By the same token, there are those who carefully avoid the pitfalls and still age—in physical terms—rapidly, despite their precautions.

One reason why some women manage to age gracefully is heredity. A smooth complexion that stays smooth at fifty, or one that becomes lined at an earlier age can be linked to the genes. Graying hair, baldness, and skin problems are only a few of the physical characteristics that are largely determined by characteristics we have inherited from our parents and ancestors.

Obviously, the woman who has inherited traits of youthful appearance has an easier time, in cosmetic terms, than the woman who has another type of genetic makeup. But the climacteric can be a time of surprises. It is perhaps fitting that during this period of physical change, the beauty problems of youth can become assets. Take, for example, the sebaceous glands. In many individuals, these glands are overactive, producing an excess of natural oils. Most commonly observed during adolescence, this excess produces a number of skin problems, clogging pores, contributing to blemishes, and causing an oily complexion. Since sebaceous glands slow production as we get older, the woman who once cursed her oily skin may later be thankful for it. No cosmetic works as well as the skin's natural oil to retard lines and wrinkles.

But sooner or later, signs of aging appear. Many people become obsessive about them, but perhaps we should consider the remarkable fact that most of what we go through in physical terms doesn't show at all. The skin has an amazing resiliency—a capacity to stretch with muscular movement, inflammation, and weight gain, and then to pull back into shape. Unfortunately this tendency diminishes with age, as the web of elastic fibrils, coiled in the *dermis* (the second, or inner layer of skin) grows less resilient.

This is not the only change in the skin. For all that has been said and written about beauty being skin deep, it must be remembered that in fact the skin is not deep at all, averaging less than five-thousandths of an inch in depth. The outer layer of skin, or epidermis, and the unseen dermis are composed of layers of cells that are constantly active. New cells are continually being formed through mitosis, the process of cell reproduction. At the same time, old cells die and gradually work their way through the layers of the skin. By the time they reach the surface of the epidermis, the process of exfoliation has been prepared to serve a new purpose. Live cells cannot live exposed to air; these dead cells on the other hand, filled with keratin (the hard substance that forms the hair and nails) that has replaced the cytoplasm or living cell matter needed for activity, now form the body's first line of defense.

Once this purpose has been served, the dead cells are sloughed off, and newer arrivals replace them.

In this way, the living skin cells are protected, while the dead cells are in effect reprogrammed to serve in the protection process.

As we age, the metabolism—or rate of body activity—slows as much as 12 percent in some individuals. In the skin, as in all other organs of the body, this gradual process is one of atrophy, shrinking, and decreased function in the cells and the structures they form. The cell also becomes weaker in its ability to use nutrients and dispose of waste matter; there is a loss of vitality.

Skin cells become dehydrated; the skin looks and feels dry and then the elastic fibrils uncoil, accompanied by a decrease in the quantity and quality of tissue support. Lines and wrinkles, sagging and drooping, are common as the skin loses some of its former resiliency.

Exfoliation slows down. Cells no longer slough off as readily as they once did, and there may be a buildup of horny tissue. Blood vessels in the skin form networks of fine lines close to the surface, which lead to increased bruising. The cells that produce melanin, the pigment that gives the skin its color, may not perform optimally; spots, blotches, and uneven coloration become more frequent.

The hair, too, changes. Growth in the hair follicle, the miniature factory where hair is produced, slows and in some cases stops. The natural coloring mechanism slows or fails, and gray hair is produced. The texture of the hair yet forming is coarser.

Toxins, poisonous substances that the body's defensive structures combat, are more easily deposited in the cells. The excretory functions slow down.

In short, the appearance changes, and the popular "young look" is more difficult to convey. The enviable woman who looked as though she spent hours in front of the mirror but who was really a "natural beauty" now has to work harder at her appearance.

The routine she follows is very important. Not only should the woman who wants to look her best take care to do what will help her, but she must avoid the things that can add to her problems. What course to pursue can be confusing, particularly when one is confronted with the endless variety of cosmetics, treatments, and devices. Skin care should be individualized, but general rules apply. Basically, a beauty program should compensate for nature's failures.

Cleanliness is always important to the skin. Yet many women, as they mature, believe that cleansing is harmful, that creaming the skin is more gentle and therefore more beneficial. The cells, however, are already lazy and benefit from stimulation.

Washing the face with a soft, clean cloth or complexion brush does more than keep the skin clean. The scrubbing action (it should be done in small, circular movements) helps to remove dead cells—an essential function now that the natural exfoliating process has slowed. In addition to removing dead cells, this movement stimulates the production of new cells and encourages cell activity, including oil production.

A soap or cleansing cream can be used, but products that have harsh detergent bases are to be avoided. Look for a mild cleansing agent, one that has a natural pH and acid/alkali balance close to that of the skin itself (the pH of the skin is normally slightly acid—pH5–6). In washing, avoid extremes of hot and cold. Water should be tepid during washing and rinsing, and a cooler, but not ice cold, rinsing can follow. Pores cannot be permanently shrunken, but a splash of cool water can temporarily close them, and can, in addition, stimulate the blood vessels to produce natural color.

Many women, especially those with oily skin, follow

cleansing with the application of an astringent or toner with an alcohol base. Alcohol, however, is a drying agent and as we get older these products are best used a drop or two at a time on a moistened cotton ball or tissue. This diluted strength will then remove excessive oil, where needed, without drying the skin unnecessarily.

Since natural hydration or moisture is not all it once was, the use of a moisturizer becomes more and more important. There are a variety of products to choose from, as every woman knows, and the choice can be confusing.

In the search for a secret ingredient that will turn back the clock, a number of discoveries have been promoted and rushed to the cosmetic counter for a day in the sun of popularity and a season at the cash register. In the past decade alone, queen bee jelly, "organic" cosmetics, hormone creams, and vitamin E preparations—among many others—have achieved fad popularity.

Considering the supposedly miraculous ingredients each has to recommend it, it's no surprise they are just that—fads—rather than permanent factors in the lives of beauty-conscious women. The extravagant claims made for queen bee jelly, for example, were disproven and recent moves toward truth-in-advertising legislation will hopefully guard against similar abuses. Organic preparations and their manufacturers are correct in claiming that many additives can be bad for the skin, and for the body as well. Yet not all organic products are necessarily good—as nonorganic preparations are not, by definition, bad.

Hormone creams, though no longer widely advertised, can be of great benefit in promoting healthy, attractive skin—particularly those containing estrogen. Unfortunately, the Food and Drug Administration must limit the amount of hormone in over-the-counter creams to insure against the side effects of excess absorption into the body of particularly sensitive women—and this limit is too low to be of much value. Stronger hormone creams used under medical supervision can, however, be beneficial.

As useless commercial hormone creams have suffered in popularity, vitamin-enriched products have grown—particularly those containing vitamin E. Perhaps it was the use of this oil-based vitamin in treating burns that started the fad. Soon, claims were being made that it could make lines disappear, cause stretch marks to vanish, and spots to fade. Unfortunately, these truths are based in a copywriter's imagination—and not in proven fact.

Which moisturizer to use? First of all think *sensibly*.

Oils and essences can be pleasing, but inevitably they add to the cost. Packaging, too, plays a role—and if you like a product's look, feel, and scent, you will feel better using it. But keep in mind that expensive is not synonymous with effective: cosmetics appeal to a number of the senses—and the sense of reason is only one.

Then think *simply*.

Water is the simplest moisturizer of all, and nature's own. Some women use an atomizer to spray a fine mist of cool water over the face frequently during the day. Try it after makeup is applied, to "set" cosmetics, and occasionally through the day to refresh the face.

Of course, water evaporates, not only from the top of the skin, but from within the cells themselves. A good moisturizer, therefore, is one that retains the water while the skin absorbs it.

Lanolin and glycerin are two such *hydrophyllic* ingredients: they promote the absorption of water. At the same time they provide a light coating on the skin that prevents evaporation. Glycerin and rosewater, a simple combination no longer as popular as it once was, is nevertheless effective. Apply as often as you like; it could hardly be less expensive.

With any moisturizer, frequent applications are a good idea. No matter how rich a cream or lotion might be, the skin will absorb only so much and no more. Apply small amounts often, rather than using (and wasting) an excessive amount once or twice a day.

Many women feel they need a heavier emollient cream. But while some of the oils from these "night cream" products actually penetrate the skin, most remain as a heavy coating. Useful under certain circumstances— skiing, for example—this coating may also clog the pores, adding more problems than it solves. Tissue off excess after a half-hour or so.

If it is essential to add moisture to the skin as we grow older, it is equally important not to dry out the skin. Who would intentionally do such a thing? The millions of women who've made the drying masks—found on cosmetic counters today—so popular.

Moisturing masks can be beneficial. "Toning" or "firming" masks, on the other hand, lend themselves to misuse. These preparations appeal, in large part, because they make the skin feel tighter—just as the beaten egg white your grandmother may have spread on her skin dried and tightened.

On balanced skins, those with enough natural moisture, these preparations are fine. But the woman with dry skin, as is so often the case during the climacteric, must remember that the tightening effect is just that: an effect. Masks do not make lines or wrinkles disappear. They do, however, make the skin drier. Check your needs carefully, or get the advice of a cosmetician who's interested in more than selling you the newest "miracle" preparation. And if you do use a toning mask or lotion, avoid areas that are constantly subject to dryness. Even the woman with a basically oily complexion must moisturize the area around the eyes and the neck.

A woman with persistent dryness problems would do well to consult her own physician. He may advise an ethical cream—one for which a prescription is necessary. These creams might contain hormones such as estrogen or cortisone. Or he may suggest a reliable over-the-counter product, but whatever his recommendation, it will be made with the individual patient in mind.

Moisturizing, cleansing, and stimulating the skin can help maintain general attractiveness, but during this time of life there may be special skin problems that require attention. It is not uncommon for a woman, at the time of the climacteric, to develop allergies and sensitivities to cosmetics—even those that she has used successfully for years.

A sudden irritation, redness, or itching may tempt a woman to apply more of the substance that causes it in an effort to conceal or soothe the problem. Keeping the possibility of an allergic reaction in mind, it is best to either stop using all cosmetics for a day or so and see if there is an improvement, or to consult a doctor immediately.

Another common problem is *keratoses*, formations of flat warty-like growths resulting from the buildup of dead cells. When the exfoliating process slows, cells are not shed quickly enough, and this type of buildup can occur, accompanied by dryness and flakiness. Pores and follicles of the skin can become clogged, inflaming glands which normally secrete through them. These growths can be easily removed in an office visit.

Some women, as they grow older, begin to notice what at first glance looks like a recurrence of adolescent acne. Red bumps and small patches develop on the face, usually around the nose and cheeks. In this disease, *acne rosacea*, the blood vessels of the skin become enlarged, accompanied by red papules and oiliness. Rosacea usually responds well to drying and antiinflammatory agents, similar to those employed in acne treatment. Cortisone and topical estrogen creams can also be effective.

Certainly no beauty problem is as closely identified with aging—or as misnamed—as so-called "liver spots." For the record, these dark spots have nothing whatever to do with the liver, but develop as a result of pigment changes in the skin. The pigment-producing mechanism, as we have discussed, can become erratic, causing spots to form. Homemade preparations have been used for centuries to fade these spots, but today chemical bleaching, or freezing and removal with liquid nitrogen or dry ice, are procedures some doctors recommend. The spots may recur, but in some cases treatment can be repeated with good cosmetic effect.

By noticing changes in the mirror and acting on what is reflected, it becomes possible to deal with problems as they develop. Changes in moles or beauty marks, particularly raised ones that become irritated, or flat blue-black growths, should be brought to the attention of a physician. These may be malignant.

If a woman doesn't have a good relationship with a dermatologist, the time of the climacteric is a good time to establish one. Changes in the skin do occur, more in some people than in others, and it can be reassuring—as well as aesthetically pleasing—to treat those that can be easily taken care of.

Some dermatologists are extremely sympathetic to the woman who is concerned with the manifestation of physical aspects of aging. Others, it must be said, treat skin disorders with great attention, but tend to wave away purely cosmetic complaints. Looking her best, I believe, is in a woman's self-interest if it is important to her, and feeling secure in one's appearance is very important—especially at a crucial time like the climacteric.

Certainly an area that should be approached from the medical, as well as cosmetic, standpoint is that of the skin and the sun. Everybody, most people would agree, looks better with a suntan. Yet excessive exposure to sunlight, particularly during its peak hours of eleven to two, can be more harmful than beneficial.

A slowly acquired suntan is all right; sunburn is bad. A sunburn is not only painful and toxic, but it damages the skin. Repeated sunburns can cause a condition known as *actinic* (or radiation) *dermatitis*—also known, for obvious reasons, as "farmer's skin" or "sailor's skin." Occurring usually in people with fair complexions, it produces symptoms that mimic those of age itself. The skin becomes dry, thin, inelastic.

Another skin condition related to sun is a type of keratoses I mentioned before. Aging skin is predisposed to keratoses of various types, and exposure to sun is the primary cause of actinic keratoses. Patches of red, slightly scaly skin appear, most often on the face and hands. And not only are they unattractive, they may be considered precancerous. This, and the growing evidence that the sun is a direct cause of other skin cancers, is reason enough to treat sunlight with respect—and caution.

How to get that "healthy" look without endangering your health? Dozens of products are available, and some actually work.

Total sunscreens—those that completely block ultraviolet rays—are recommended for problem exposure areas, such as the nose or shoulders. These products generally include the oxides of zinc or titanium, or benzophenones among their listed ingredients.

Partial sunscreens attempt to permit passage of tanning rays while blocking out those that merely burn. Ingredients to look for are glyceryl para-aminobenzoate, or any of the benzophenones, cinnamates, or anthanilates. Don't attempt to remember (or even pronounce!) them all; just take along a list the next time you're shopping for a suntan preparation.

And keep in mind that the sun may be drying skin already dehydrated. Follow your suntan sprees with a good moisturizer.

Of course the look of a suntan can come, today, from a bottle or tube—along with a few other looks, some good, some foolish.

While writing this chapter, I attended a dinner party and saw a walking example of what not to do in terms of makeup. A woman was present—a television executive—whose age I later learned was forty-five. She had apparently decided to compensate for age with quantity rather than quality. Overpainted almost beyond imagination, she looked like a caricature of the youthful look she was struggling to achieve. In addition, I wondered how the heavy makeup—more suited to a television studio than an intimate setting—might further aggravate her troubles by blocking and clogging her pores.

Certainly makeup needs are individualized, and an aesthetician or cosmetologist is best qualified to advise on personal cosmetic problems. Yet as a physician who sees dozens of women regularly, I've noticed that a few general rules apply.

Begin at the beginning: for dry skins, an oil-based foundation may be best—and why not apply a moisturizer ten minutes or so before the foundation. If skin is oily, or if a tendency toward rosacea or similar problems has been noted, a less oily base should be used. And remember that in choice of foundations, color plays a key role; a warmer tone can compensate for a lack in natural tonal warmth.

After the foundation comes the most common makeup mistake of all: the use of concealer sticks or creams under the eye. Lighter than the foundation tone, they are a popular attempt to hide sags and circles. But unless carefully blended with the foundation, such attempts can actually call more attention to the problem, rather than minimize it. Using a darker shadow on the eyelid, an actress patient of mine pointed out, is a much better way to distract an observer from under-eye problems.

The "concealer" theory became popular several years ago as part of the "contour" makeup concept. Using light and dark creams to shade and highlight the skin is an art, and at its best can be very effective. But in unskilled hands, this approach to makeup is far from flattering. Some women fail to realize a simple fact: there is only so much that makeup can do. Assets can be played up, and problems played down. But a more natural look is preferable to something stagy and artificial—and at last is fashionable as well.

Soft, natural lines are flattering, particularly as we get older. Dramatic sweeps of very dark eyeliners can give the face a hard look, especially when combined with overtweezed eyebrows and an overdramatic hairstyle. Some women like this look; others must not be aware of the full effect they create at their makeup table.

The use of lipstick is a good example of this confusion. As tiny lines begin to develop around the mouth, many women appear to believe that a swath of bright color across—and often around—the lips will solve the problem. And, of course, this only serves to call attention to the mouth *and* its wrinkles. Choose a neutral shade instead, preferably one with moisturizing ingredients that can help the problem, not add to it.

And no matter what makeup you use, never make the mistake of trying to conceal irritations or rashes in the hope they will go away. Many such blemishes may disappear on their own—but not under a constant coating of makeup, which can aggravate even the most minor skin problems. Check them with your physician or dermatologist.

As you think of what goes on your face, consider what you rub your face against. Avoid overly starched pillow cases that can chafe and irritate the skin, and watch for harsh bleaches or laundering agents that can leave a residue unless fully rinsed. This goes for towels and facecloths, too; like pillow cases, they should be changed frequently, if not daily.

Applying makeup is an art; removing it is equally important. Makeup removal, like all cleansing, should be followed with a moisturizer.

In addition to cosmetics, some women try improving the appearance with various exercises and "toning" devices. Facial exercise is widely touted by those who specialize in it as a business, and expertly directed it may have positive results. Do-it-yourself attempts, at least those that I have seen (and I've made it my business to observe several patients and their results), do not seem effective. Chin straps, likewise, may be overvalued: the muscles of the chin come to rely on this support, which is not, obviously, worn during the day. Facial massage, by hand or machine, should be administered by a professional. Amateur attempts may aggravate skin problems, and if done too earnestly, can break blood vessels.

The hair—in terms of color, condition, and style—should blend with the face for a total, flattering image. Yet, like the skin, the hair changes.

Just as the facial skin often becomes sensitive during the climacteric, the scalp does the same. It is possible, and not uncommon, to develop allergies to bleaches and coloring products that have been used for years without any problem, and the patch tests recommended by hair-coloring manufacturers should be made before *each* application.

Admittedly, many women don't do this, nor do all beauty operators, and I've had patients phone from the beauty parlor in a panic at a sudden reddening or itching. When this happens, stop the color treatment at once. Wash the hair and the skin (both face and scalp) and immediately seek medical advice. The bleaching and coloring process may not be completed, but "waiting it out" and following through despite an allergy can cause long-term discoloration or other problems.

Patients often ask how frequently the hair should be washed. There is no hard-and-fast rule except as often as necessary for the feel and look you want. It is not so much how often you shampoo as how you shampoo and what you use that matters. Use a mild preparation—not a harsh detergent. Balance is the key word, as it is in facial soaps.

Keep dandruff under control. Not only do its white flakes detract from the appearance of the hair, it can develop into a dermatitis of the scalp. There are several good medicinal shampoos that used once or twice a month will prevent this irritating and ugly condition.

Never rub too hard, and don't believe that the more shampoo you use the better your hair will look. Instead, I recommend a single, gentle lathering, and avoiding pulling the hair. When it is wet, the porous hair shaft absorbs water and stretches—it can be, and too often is, literally pulled out of shape.

Rinse thoroughly to remove residue from shampoo, and rinse both the hair and the scalp. Just as a moisturizer is used on the face, a conditioner can be used on the hair with good results in terms of appearance and manageability. Follow directions carefully, and bear in mind that no matter how good a conditioner is, hair will absorb only so much and no more. Rinse well (unless the product you use is intended to be left on), since too much conditioner can make the hair gummy and dull-looking.

During the climacteric, there is a general tendency toward thinning hair. The hair root, in addition, may become weak. Avoid rollers rolled too tightly (never sleep on them), and excessive brushing (a hundred strokes can do more harm than fabled good, particularly at this time of life).

The natural oils that moisturize the face also moisturize the scalp, and through the hair follicle, they coat the hair shaft providing natural shine and luster. As the oil supply decreases, breakage and split ends are more common. Using a warm air setting on the hair dryer, rather than hot, is important. Also essential is guarding against the effects of heat and wind. Wear a scarf or, preferably, a hat on the beach or when in heavy sunlight. If you swim in the ocean, or in a chemically treated pool, wash hair as soon as possible to remove sea salts, minerals, and chemicals from hair and scalp.

Today wigs and hairpieces are increasingly popular. As long as they are made on a base that allows the hair and scalp to breathe, they aren't harmful. Many women wear stretch wigs. Others wear wigs or hairpieces that must be fastened to the hair. If you wear this type of hairpiece, be sure to avoid the mistake of fastening it day after day in the same place. This repeated stress on a single area of the hair can cause a thin spot.

As a woman ages, she may be tempted to restore the natural color of the hair she had in her youth. Nothing (providing you have no allergy or sensitivity to the product used) is wrong with coloring the hair, but from a cosmetic standpoint it is better to select a color that is lighter than natural. Black or dark brown hair accentuates facial sag, and makes a harsh frame for lines and wrinkles. A lighter color is far more flattering.

And please remember the good sense I recommended for facial care. There are few if any genuine "miracles" for turning back the clock—for the complexion or for the hair. It's true that experiments have linked vitamin B6 to hair color in mice; mice deprived of this nutrient grayed. From time to time, as these experiments are publicized, drugstores are suddenly besieged by people buying B6 (and every other B vitamin) in the false hope that gray hair would turn back to its natural color. I'm afraid that gray hair, when it comes, is the natural color—and the decision to keep it gray or not is an individual matter.

The only miracle for aging skin or hair—and for the other changes of the climacteric—is nature's own: estrogen.

And that brings us back to the story of Janet Milam. Within a week of her confrontation with the mirror, Janet Milam consulted me for the symptoms she had discovered. Though hardly severe, they were adversely affecting all aspects of her life. A petite woman, attractively and very stylishly attired, she conveyed the impression of a sophisticated pixie. It was easy to recognize that she was a woman experienced in self-control. But her eyes and voice betrayed tinges of panic.

She had moved to New York from South Carolina three years earlier to work for a dress designer. Her work had been good, and she was in line for a promotion. She was proud of her success as a career woman.

Her social life had also been satisfying. Arthur was an attentive lover and she had an interesting group of friends. There was only one problem: her true age was becoming harder to conceal.

In her personal life, Janet's "white lie" had posed no problem. Arthur had never questioned her age; he had always been attracted to older women, and even at her false age of thirty-eight he was three years her junior. As for Janet, aside from an occasional realization that she could literally be a younger friend's mother, she felt very much at ease doing whatever they did.

But for the last few months she had found a day at the office increasingly trying. She was tired all the time, she told me, and every few days some new minor symptoms would appear to replace the ones that had gone away. She began refusing social invitations under the pretext of work she had to do at home. And though she felt an increasing need to be with Arthur, she found herself rejecting him sexually, to the point that he was becoming impatient. Her health, Janet feared, was going to cause her to lose both her job and her lover.

Furthermore, she was becoming frightened to look in the mirror and had to control a tendency to use too much makeup. She was going to the hairdresser more frequently, watching her diet more closely, and being careful not to complain when someone asked her how she felt. She also had to be careful not to be caught off guard, because she had noticed that whenever she thought she was alone she involuntarily let her face and posture collapse.

Besides the signs of anxiety and depression, she was having headaches, trouble with her eyes, constipation, insomnia, sore gums, rushes of warm tinglings in her skin, and irregular menses. Hesitantly she voiced her concern that some of these symptoms might be related to the menopause.

She had last had a physical three years earlier when she had joined the New York company. She had felt in perfect health, and everything on the examination had been normal. She didn't feel in perfect health now; she felt miserable. She wanted a complete examination and my opinion about some rejuvenating injections a popular magazine had reported were being given by a doctor in Los Angeles with miraculous results. If I thought they were effective, she was willing to fly out there to get them.

A week later, when I discussed with her the results of the examination, I could report several things worthy of comment. The pain in her gums was due to infected wisdom teeth. The fatigue and insomnia were symptoms of her anxiety and depression. She had two problems with her eyes. Her near vision was poor because she had presbyopia, an inescapable consequence of aging. The lens loses its elasticity so that it can no longer focus clearly on near objects. She also had a mild conjunctivitis that could be due to an allergy to her makeup, an irritation from polluted air, or possibly a nonspecific inflammation that sometimes comes with advancing years.

Janet looked older than her stated age by a few years, but much younger than her actual age. Her skin still had turgor and resiliency, and her body tone and contours were those of a younger woman. The most important thing was her Estrogen Index. It wasn't extraordinarily low, but in view of the peculiar sensations she had noted in her skin, which could reflect incipient flushes, her estrogen supply was probably insufficient. This, in addition to her headaches, constipation, and lack of sense of well-being, could represent a premenopausal or early climacteric state.

"I know you are telling me that medically there is nothing seriously wrong. But I think you can appreciate the significance of what you are saying. I can't say I'm happy to have my suspicions confirmed. What about my ovaries? Does that mean I can't have a baby?"

"I doubt if you are ovulating, or if you are, it is only sporadic. Your menses are too irregular."

"That's a blow," she sighed. "I don't think I ever really

wanted a child until this moment, now you tell me I can't have one. That puts me in a rather peculiar position with Arthur. I'm not sure how he would feel. It's certainly a problem I've got to think about. But outside of that, the ovaries are not all that important to good health, are they?"

"The ovaries aren't, no. But their hormones are. Estrogen can be as essential to the body as insulin. But an adequate supply can be furnished pharmacologically."

"That's some consolation," Janet said.

She then asked about the rejuvenating injections she had read about. I had investigated them after her first visit. The theory sounded good—giving aging cells new life by providing them with a generous supply of the basic materials of which they are composed; a ramification, or diluted version, of cellular therapy, which is not recognized in the United States. But I could find nothing about them reported in the medical literature, and none of my colleagues knew anything of them.

"I think you should forget it for the moment," I told her. "Wait for some follow-up information. Perhaps you can even find someone who has tried it. Then you can make up your mind. If it works, it can rejuvenate your cells in a few years as well as it can now."

"So if that's out of the window, what do you suggest?" Janet asked. "I know I've got to feel better. I can't neglect my work or my boyfriend much longer and get away with it."

"To begin with I would suggest ERT," I told her. "I'm sure the hormones will make you feel better, get rid of most of your annoying symptoms. Also attending to those infected teeth will eliminate a source of toxicity and improve your general health. Your psychological state needs some special attention. In the first place, no one can function properly without adequate sleep. Nor can anyone attend to his business and personal obligations if anxiety is always distracting his thoughts or because depression converts constructive thinking to worry, his mind going around in a circle.

"Psychotrophic drugs, such as sleeping pills, tranquilizers, stimulants, etc., should not become a way of life, but like antibiotics there is a time when they are necessary. Once you feel better physically, more than likely you can cope with your petulant psyche. But as you pointed out, you have some problems that need immediate attention. So I suggest that you take two of these tranquilizers at bedtime. The immediate effect will let you sleep, and a weaker effect, that is prolonged into the next day, will help you to deal with your anxiety. If the anxiety seems to be building up, break a tablet in half and take it."

Janet had another question. "What about the way I look?" she asked. "In the fashion business the women have to have the vibrations and figure of a twenty-year-old. I've come to think that doing a good job is only peripheral. I've seen in the few years I've been there several very competent women put out to pasture because people began to notice their age, the crow's-feet around their eyes, the frown wrinkles, the bulging around the waist. One of them had three children to support. I thought about plastic surgery. . . ."

"You don't need it now," I assured her.

"Even if I did, I would be crazy to have it. Someone would surely find out, and that would be the end of Janet Milam, fashion expert. And then there's my weight. I know I'm at least six or seven pounds too heavy."

I disagreed, at least in part. "By health statistics, no; for your job, maybe yes. Once you are in a better frame of mind you can take them off. It is basically a matter of self-discipline, and you seem to have an adequate supply of that. As a start forget about all starches and sweets. If that doesn't work, we can think about giving you an appetite suppressant. It may help control your appetite but you can't totally rely on it.

"Losing weight is only part of making the body look good. You've also got to firm it up. With age, the muscles and the tissues under the skin lose their tone. Part of the subcutaneous tissue is fat and when a woman sheds pounds, the skin tends to become loose. Exercise is the best thing to compensate for these changes.

"I'll give you an outline of a simple routine," I told her. "It just takes fifteen minutes a day and is relatively unoffensive. Get it over and done with in the morning. It may be a bore, but when you finish you'll feel better both physically and mentally, and it won't increase your appetite."

"And my skin? . . ." she asked.

"It's on your side—figuratively speaking. I don't know whether it's your genes or what, but for your age it is in good condition."

"But lately I've noticed it is a bit dry, especially on my face, the back of my hands, and my arms."

"Then I can suggest something for you. To reinforce the hydrating effect the oral estrogens are going to have, use this cream with estrogen to get a concentrated effect where it is most needed. It also contains a small amount of cortisone to counteract any inflammations. In the future you may have to work a little harder and try some new things. As for your makeup and your clothes, you have proved that you know what is right for you. That sense of intuition, not some rebellious itch, will continue to guard you from stepping out of the limits of good taste and inviting criticism."

"And how should I deal with Arthur?" Janet asked.

This time I had no prescription. "That's a problem you are going to have to work out for yourself."

Janet Milam came back every three or four weeks for about eight months, though I had told her earlier she needn't see me that frequently. During that period she rarely had any physical complaint; her Estrogen Index returned to normal; she lost weight; she adjusted to the bifocal contact lenses; she had several changes in hair styles; and she always had on a new and attractive outfit. She still liked her work, always had some new interest to report, and was still involved with Arthur. I seemed to sense, however, a hint of apprehension.

If she were anxious, I could understand it. I compare her in my mind to a matador, repeatedly exposing herself with bravura to a fatal attack. Anxiety is a natural consequence of this constant vulnerability. Besides the real pressures in her life, something deeper seemed to be bothering her, and on one visit she confided a desire to make a change in her life, to reorganize it in some way so she would feel more secure.

I saw her next for her semiannual checkup, and then, several months later, Janet Milam came in to see me for the last time. She looked exceptionally well, and I told her so.

"Thank you," she said as she sat back in the chair in a relaxed manner I had never observed in her before. "And I feel great."

"Then what are you here for?" I joked.

"To tell you good-bye. I'm leaving New York, going back to South Carolina."

"Do you have a new job?" She shook her head. "Retiring?" I asked.

"Oh, I'm not giving up. By no means. You could say I'm just starting, taking on a new life. And I might be biting off more than I can chew. But at least I won't be living a lie, walking a tightrope day after day, night after night. I could have managed it for a few years longer, but after that I wasn't so sure. I know I still look much younger than I am, and I feel younger than I look. Still, any way I look at it, I'm not young. And I'm tired of having to pretend I am. I'll be fifty next week.

"No," Janet continued, smiling now, "I'm leaving the company. And I'm going to be a mother."

Janet laughed at my shocked expression.

"Now, don't look so surprised, Doctor," she said. "I'm going to be the mother of a ready-made family."

Janet was quick to fill me in on the details. She'd gone to South Carolina on company business, and met a widower with three children. The relationship had blossomed during several visits, and when the man proposed to Janet on a trip to New York, she accepted.

"He's not as handsome as Arthur," Janet told me. "But he's kind, decisive, responsible, reliable, and hardworking. He's financially secure, and he knows my real age and loves me. The children like me, too. So off I go—I'm going to be a housewife in a small southern town, and I'm going to like it. And you know what the best part is?"

"What?" I asked, sincerely pleased for her.

"For the first time in my life I'm going to have the pleasure of hearing people say, 'But you don't look anywhere near your age!' "

She left my office, an attractive and happy woman. As a physician, I knew that treating Janet's physical problems had helped her through the crisis of self-realization. Her attractiveness, however, something she had been so afraid of losing, wasn't all due to any prescription. Janet *felt* attractive.

Free of the pressure of keeping up and living a lie, and able to accept herself, she was more relaxed and better able to come to terms with her own identity as a human being.

She could look in the mirror—and instead of facing a crisis, she could face the reflection of the woman she wanted to be.

More Than Skin Deep

Cosmetic Surgery, Diet, and Exercise

Growing older gracefully is an attitude as much as a physical process.

We admire—and at times envy—the man or woman who wears his or her years well. Such a person seems generously gifted by nature with some secret endowment we can see but can't quite define. As a result, we often mistake a positive mental attitude for "good genes." Heredity, as we've discussed, plays an important role in physical appearance, but the person who wants to find fault with his looks can do so no matter how slowly he seems to age.

Very few of us, of course, would consciously choose to concentrate on our liabilities rather than our assets, but often in the turmoil that can be part of the transition to the middle years, graying hair or facial lines can become focal points for a variety of physical and mental complaints that can be temporarily overwhelming.

Sadly, many doctors tend to minimize the cosmetic aspects of this time of life. They may be well-intentioned, thinking in terms of crowded appointment books and their patients' well-being and trying to find a balance. Health, the physician may reason, is all that matters. How a patient looks, unless his appearance is symptomatic of a specific disease, simply isn't important.

A man or a woman concerned about appearance is obviously going to feel differently. Conditioned, however, to the medical profession's oversight of cosmetic problems, the patient who would like to talk with a doctor about looks often doesn't dare to mention the subject. The patient may even begin to wonder if this interest in how one looks isn't obsessive and unhealthy!

In most cases, one needn't plague oneself with such doubts. Care about how we look is normal and healthy— it's the kind of concern that shows an involvement with life, a desire to participate in the world and to function in society.

Later in this chapter I want to spend a good deal of time discussing cosmetic surgery, because it's a complex and timely subject. But for the moment I want to concentrate on the simple things. Think of yourself as an automobile. You should be working with your doctor on the care of the engine and vital parts—but why don't you take a minute to think about the scratched fenders and rusted bumpers time has left you with. Go through the list of corns, broken teeth, and blemishes. Now, how about your nails? How long has it been since they've been given some real attention? Meanwhile, don't forget about your toenails; perhaps you won't be going about without shoes as often as your son or daughter, but that's no reason to ignore them—especially the nails on the little toes, always a problem.

And lose that weight! Don't think of yourself as one of those lumbering Cadillacs of the fifties, but rather as a newer, sleeker model popular since "energy crisis" became part of our vocabulary. For the energy crisis is just as applicable to our own bodies. Who has the energy to waste carrying around an extra twenty—or even ten—pounds?

You may find yourself with a weight problem now where one never existed before, but that's no excuse to pretend it doesn't exist. Watch your diet carefully—with food prices what they've become, you should be doing it anyway! The first time you find yourself struggling with a zipper that just won't close, do something about it.

On the subject of clothes, remember that "stylish" doesn't necessarily mean "trendy." Clothes that look terrific on some young boy or half-starved model aren't always right for you. If the fashion of the moment doesn't suit you, be self-assured enough to wear what does. Be comfortable—not sloppy—and let your own good judgment, not a fashion magazine, be your guide.

"Good judgment," I know, sounds awfully vague. Perhaps there are men and women who truly have no sense of what is attractive for them, but I suspect they are rare. More likely, they have a sense that tells them what's right and wrong. But they just don't listen. Maybe they rationalize that they are being strong and brave enough to look the way they like, fanciful. But they fool only themselves.

If you ever feel unsure of yourself, just picture in your mind a contemporary you admire. No doubt he or she is well-groomed, dresses stylishly, not flamboyantly, and doesn't try to look inappropriately young or unnecessarily old. And one thing, I suspect, is certain: there is a pride of carriage.

Good posture is essential, now more than ever. A lifetime of poor habits must now be changed. Not only is bad posture unattractive, it's unhealthy. Proper posture puts the weight on the skeleton, not on the muscles. Many of the backaches and muscle pains associated with middle age are a direct result of poor posture.

More than simple posture, all of your body movements should come under close scrutiny at this time of life. "Body language" has become a popular subject, and you owe it to yourself to see what your body is "saying." Walking, sitting, talking—be aware of your body movements, and take care that they present you in the most flattering light possible. Don't be apologetic in your movement; keep erect, be assertive. And watch those mannerisms! Flirtatious movements of the head and hands may not be as attractive as they once were. If you're one of those people who "talk with their hands," be careful not to overdo it—you don't want people to be so caught up watching your busy hands that they don't hear what you're saying.

Speaking of body language, you're likely to become more aware of how the wear and tear of time has imposed certain restrictions on muscular strength and joint mobility. It's true that you're not as flexible or as quick as you used to be, and you want to take it easy on strenuous work or exercise. Always take care not to exceed your physical limitations. But at the same time you don't want to give in to physical deterioration. Don't let a little arthritis confine you to an armchair, or your fear of a heart attack cause you to shuffle about like a ninety-year-old.

After taking careful stock of yourself and your cosmetic problems, you might find that you can accept the facts of your appearance—changes included—with no serious problem of adjustment. If, on the other hand, the sight of a double chin or deep facial lines is something you just can't live with, the time has come when you may not have to.

Peace of mind, it's often said, cannot be bought. It is, however, possible to "buy" a degree of outward self-assurance—at least to the extent that you can feel more at peace with the face you see reflected in the mirror.

I'm speaking, of course, about cosmetic surgery.

Much has been said and written about the various reconstructive approaches to beauty. Yet very few people have a true understanding of the subject. Their information (and misinformation) comes from popular magazines, the gossip columns, and the latest rumors floating around the bridge table and the golf course.

When we think or talk about plastic surgery, for example, we tend to think in terms of extremes. The movie star or acquaintance, for example, who has had this type of procedure done looks either "wonderful" or "terrible" depending on the success of the surgery and our point of view. Most patients, when they discuss the subject with me, and presumably with their friends, talk about "complete face lifts," and more and more frequently the body and face lift that is often referred to as "the complete overhaul."

General ideas of what cosmetic surgery costs, of what it can and cannot do, and of what it entails as a procedure are often far off target in terms of fact.

Perhaps the greatest misconception of all is that the most successful cosmetic surgery is the most obvious. Nothing could be further from the truth. The best cosmetic surgery results in a generally improved appearance. Your family and closest friends may actually see the specific change, but others—including friends and relatives who don't know the details of your surgery—should be able to tell only that you look better.

Very few things are less attractive than the taut expressionless face of a man or woman whose cosmetic surgeon worked not too wisely, but too well! Increasingly, doctors and patients alike are looking to smaller-scale procedures, done as necessary.

What this means in practical terms is that there is no need to wait until you feel you need a total face lift before looking into cosmetic surgery. This is an outdated attitude, but one that still prevails.

Not long ago, an attractive patient of mine, an executive with a major public relations firm, sat in my office, complaining about the bags under her eyes and her sagging lids. I had to agree that this problem made her look older than she was, and that her eyes, as she put it, seemed "ten years older than the rest of my face."

I couldn't, however, go along with the solution she proposed. Sighing, she told me that she'd wait a few years until the rest of her face "really started to go," and then check in for a face lift using several weeks of vacation time to recover.

My patient was surprised, and pleased, to learn that there was no need to wait. Her eyes were her problem; in time, she might become displeased with a sagging chin or a wrinkled complexion, but in the meantime, she could have her eyes taken care of with no need of several weeks for recuperation.

I told my patient that it was possible to check into a hospital the evening before surgery and leave a day or two later. What's more, she could be back at work the next week with sunglasses masking discoloration. A month after our talk, she was back in my offices, singing the praise of her cosmetic surgeon.

"It was so much easier than I thought," she told me. "All it took, really, was a long weekend. And look at me now, Dr. Parrish."

I looked, and gave her my hearty approval. If I hadn't been the doctor she'd spoken with about the operation, I'd only have known that she looked more rested and attractive than she'd appeared in some time.

A growing number of cosmetic surgeons are doing eye

lifts and other procedures on an out-patient basis. This practice has reached its height not in our own country, but in Japan, where cosmetic surgery is done almost on an assembly-line basis. Naturally, an office visit is less costly than a hospital stay. As a result, it is possible to have an eye lift in Japan for as little as $150, as opposed to the $750 to $1,500 one might pay in America.

Don't think, however, as a patient of mine did, that by going to Japan you can get a beautifying operation and a vacation for the price you'd pay for surgery alone in this country. As I told my patient, cosmetic surgery is surgery nonetheless. Complications can arise—and being thousands of miles from your doctor is no bargain when you need him.

In counseling patients who are considering cosmetic surgery, I recommend sticking as close to home as possible. Many people feel that procedures of this type must be kept secret for some reason. Certainly there is nothing to be ashamed of in wanting to look one's best, and traveling hundreds or thousands of miles to have an operation "on the QT" is ridiculous.

A reputable cosmetic surgeon will want to see his patients before and after surgery as well as in the operating room. This is essential for both his benefit and the patient's.

In this, as in any type of surgery, it is necessary for doctor and patient to communicate. The doctor must fully understand what kind of result the patient is expecting from the surgery. The patient, by the same token, must know what can and cannot be achieved. If a man or woman thinks in terms of "looking twenty years younger" after such an operation, he or she is bound to be disappointed. The patient must realize the limitations of surgery as well as the potential for success.

Very often, the patient who is thinking about cosmetic surgery will consult the same doctor a friend or acquaintance went to. This can work out well—providing you and your friend have the same temperament. When patients ask my advice, I try to give them the names of several surgeons whose work I'm familiar with. But whether they plan to consult a doctor I've recommended or someone they've heard about from a friend, I advise them to take their time, be selective.

During the course of one's life, there are bound to be health crises where there is no time or opportunity to select a surgeon. If you have appendicitis, your chief concern is having your appendix out; there isn't time to see if you are compatible with the man who performs the operation.

Cosmetic surgery is different. There is time to consider and choose. Since the success of the operation will depend on your rapport with your doctor as well as his skill, it's worth taking all the time you need to find the right man.

What qualities should you look for in a cosmetic surgeon? The answer is very simple: those qualities that help you to feel at ease with him. Patience, an openness of communication, and a willingness to explain the procedure to be followed and to answer all your questions—these are important. Your doctor should point out risks involved and any potential problems that might result.

Above all, your doctor should be interested in you as a person, rather than just as a prospective client. Most cosmetic surgeons are dedicated professionals in every sense of the word. Occasionally, however, a doctor may be overzealous, letting his own enthusiasm sway a patient's decision. If, after talking with a cosmetic surgeon, you want more time to make your decision or to get another opinion, take it; don't feel pressured.

What can you expect after you've found the right doctor?

The first step, obviously, is to decide just what is to be

done. You will undoubtedly have your own ideas about what is "wrong" with the way you look, but you should keep an open mind. After all, the surgeon brings to your case the benefit of his extensive training and his experience with numerous patients before you.

Let me cite an example. A few years ago, a patient of mine asked me to refer her to a cosmetic surgeon. Her problem was a common one—the "turkey wattle," or excess skin hanging from chin to neck. In her late forties, my patient told me that she was satisfied with the rest of her appearance. She didn't feel she needed a face lift, she just wanted something done about this specific problem.

The doctor she consulted agreed, but he also suggested that her prominent nose be reduced and refined. She came back to my office to get my opinion, and to express hers.

"I've lived with this nose of mine for forty-eight years," she said. "I was never a beauty contest winner, Dr. Parrish. Now the plastic surgeon wants me to have a nose job!"

For my own information as well as the patient's, I called the surgeon and talked about the case. His feeling was that a slight refinement would greatly improve my patient's total appearance, and that since she would be in the hospital for her chin correction, the time would be opportune. The doctor explained to me, as he had to her, that he wasn't suggesting a nose "bob" or anything akin to it. The slightest refinement, he explained, was all that was needed.

My patient gave the matter some more thought, and when her surgeon showed her two identical medical photographs of her profile, one retouched to approximate the results of surgery, she agreed.

The result was excellent. Not only was her turkey wattle gone, but her new nose was a subtle, flattering improvement. It was still strong, but instead of having a downward hook, it was straight. As a result, her face didn't seem pulled downward; the under-eye area wasn't as prominent as it had been.

"You know," she said, "the other night I had dinner with a cousin who I grew up with. She told me how well I looked, and she didn't even know I'd had anything done to my nose. And Dr. Parrish, it couldn't have been just my chin—I was wearing a turtleneck because it was so cold out."

Medical photographs, which the surgeon uses as a guide, can be very useful in letting patients see approximately what can be done surgically. If you decide to pursue the possibilities of such an operation, your doctor will no doubt send you for a full set of photographs. (If you are overweight he will probably insist on a weight loss first.) Be prepared: The photographs are certain to be the most unflattering you've ever had taken! The photographer isn't at all interested in making you look your best. The lighting and angles used do just the opposite.

Your doctor will probably sketch on one or more of the photos (or use a retouching paint to simulate) the postsurgical result he wants to achieve. He may, instead, use only sketches. The surgeon or his nurse will take a medical history, and it is most important for you to answer the questions in detail. Don't forget to give him a complete list of the medications you may be taking for any reason.

When you decide to go ahead with your surgery, plan for your recovery as well. You may have to wait for weeks or even months for your appointment; if you're planning to have something of this sort done during a vacation, start making plans well in advance, preferably several months ahead.

Swelling and discoloration are common with cosmetic surgery. Rest can help to minimize them. Most cosmetic surgeons I know advise their patients to take it as easy as possible both before and after their operation. Resting before your operation will build up your reserve of strength. After surgery, you won't be looking your best and will have to go through a recovery period. Well-meaning friends can do more for you by staying away than by visiting, and you'll do yourself a favor if you so advise them.

As for the operation itself, that depends on just what you're having done and on the doctor who is doing it. It's probable that you'll be asked to check into the hospital a day or so before your surgery is scheduled, and that you'll have basic tests and a chest X-ray. The surgery itself is relatively painless (the choice of a local or general anesthetic depends on what you are having done and your general health). Every effort will be made to keep you as comfortable as possible after surgery, and your cooperation and close adherence to your doctor's advice will help assure success.

More and more people are having cosmetic surgery, yet it must be remembered that there are some who are not good candidates for such operations. If you are in poor general health, or if you have a condition that complicates surgery or endangers your health, then you will be advised against it. If you are prone to keloids (raised scar tissue) solving one cosmetic problem can create another; therefore certain procedures may not be for you.

A good cosmetic surgeon will consider your needs, your facial structure, and your general health in counseling you, and this expert advice is essential to a successful result.

He will also help to clear up any misconceptions you

may have about cosmetic surgery in general. And when it comes to the numerous procedures that can be used to improve the appearance, an expert is definitely needed.

The man or woman who is considering having cosmetic work done must be aware that in medicine, as in every other field of work, there are a few individuals who are more interested in their bank accounts than in their patients. This small but frightening group includes those who promise "miracles," and whose methods may not only be unorthodox, but damaging.

Several years ago, the widespread use of silicone injections was being touted as a major breakthrough in the medical world's approach to cosmetic improvement. Liquid silicone was used to enlarge breasts, to "fill" wrinkles in the forehead and on the upper lip, and to accentuate the cheekbones.

Injections were often massive—and it was only months and years later that some patients found themselves in serious trouble. Many women who had had their busts enlarged via silicone noticed a hardening of the substance, a danger sign which, fortunately, many reported to their physicians. In some cases, the silicone was easily removed. In others, including those that had been neglected, cancer of the breast was found, and a mastectomy was necessary for the patient's survival.

The use of silicone in the face posed its own problems. People who had had their cheekbones "built up" via silicone shots woke up weeks, months, or years after the treatment, and found that the substance that was supposed to have adhered to bone had shifted. The lumps of silicone traveled to other parts of the face and body, posed very serious problems, and necessitated removal.

It is true that while federal authorities in America have restricted the use of silicone sharply, its use in other countries is widespread. It's true, also, that some of this contraband liquid silicone makes its way into the hands of unscrupulous physicians (and nonprofessional quacks) who use it indiscriminately. Some go so far as to use a form of liquid silicone manufactured for industrial use on human patients, promising miraculous changes, but actually posing grave health problems.

Silicone, current studies indicate, can be useful, and it has a future in cosmetic treatment. At present, a small number of doctors have official sanction to experiment with liquid silicone, which they use in far smaller amounts and with much greater care than was done at first by those who too quickly seized what appeared to be a wonder treatment.

Silicone gel is another matter entirely. It is used in an encased form for implantation in cosmetic surgery, balancing areas of the face (the chin, very commonly, is built up in this way) and the body (the surgical implantation of this form of silicone is used in the breasts) with good, safe results.

If a doctor recommends silicone for you, be sure to get all the facts about the type of silicone he is referring to, and the possible dangers.

Another form of treatment that can be effective and safe if done by a competent professional, but which is very dangerous in the hands of lay "experts," is chemical peeling of the skin. By itself or in connection with full or partial face lifts, chemical peeling can reduce fine wrinkles (on the upper lip, for example), scars or pits, and some discoloration of the skin. It is particularly useful for removing hyperpigmented areas, as well as fine wrinkling of the hands, the most telltale part of our body.

A very strong chemical, often phenol or trichloracetic acid, is used to burn off the top layer of skin. After application, the face may be covered with adhesive tape for a day or two. The chemical produces a burn, and once the tape is removed (chemical powders are applied at this time) a hard crust begins to form. Within a week or so, this falls away, and a "new" skin is revealed. Liquid nitrogen and fluorouracil are used for spot peeling and the removal of certain skin cancers.

These are effective procedures for certain people, but they don't work for everyone. Some discomfort is inevitable, and even after the procedure is completed, one must follow carefully instructions about avoiding sun and using only cosmetics approved by the doctor—often over a period of several months.

Not every woman is an ideal candidate for this procedure, known as *chemosurgery*. Skin type, individual biochemistry, and health considerations are very important here. Generally speaking, lighter-skinned individuals are the best candidates. The darker the complexion, the more conspicuous the boundary line between treated and untreated skin after chemosurgery.

Tragically, many lay practitioners of chemical peeling promise success to every unfortunate woman who crosses their path, without informing her of the dangers inherent or of the fact that chemical peeling is a medical procedure that can be legally done only by the profession.

The government has cracked down on these lay practitioners, and continues to do so, but some still operate under the cover of secrecy. In their hands, a chemical peel can be disfiguring and dangerous. Some of these people administer a very mild face peel that may not be as harmful, but that outside chance isn't worth the risk, so avoid it.

Another process that is used to remove fine wrinkles, blemishes, and discolorations is *dermabrasion*. The doctor uses a high-speed brush of wire to literally rub out problem areas. The skin is denuded down to its raw basal layer, over which a crusty scab forms. When it falls away, new skin is revealed. Once again, the patient must follow guidelines about sun and cosmetics, as well as skin type and coloring.

Obviously, any type of cosmetic surgery is an expense, both in terms of time and money. Costs vary depending on what is done, and doctors have their own individual fee schedules. In considering cosmetic surgery, be sure to find out if the form of health and hospital insurance you carry will help defray some of the cost. Many such plans do not extend to operations and procedures undertaken for purely cosmetic purposes.

Remember, too, that what can be done to the face can, in many cases, be done for the body as well. Breast lifts, buttock lifts, thigh reductions and the like are being done more and more often, mostly for actresses, socialites, and those in the public eye.

It is essential to remember that no form of cosmetic surgery is permanent. Lines in the face aren't determined by nature at random. Facial expressions, which all of us have, play a part in setting them. A woman who has a complete face lift may, immediately after the operation, find her "laugh lines" gone. In time, assuming she's going to laugh and smile, they will return. Excess skin can be trimmed by the surgeon, but that does not mean that the new face will last forever. The loss of elasticity is inevitable and ongoing, especially when there is an estrogen deficiency. Face-lifting deals with the situation at hand and treats it cosmetically, but it does not and cannot stop the aging process.

Many people who have cosmetic surgery find that within five to ten years they want another operation. That doesn't mean the procedure is addictive—it simply means they like the results.

If you are considering cosmetic surgery, there are several good books on the subject. Among them, Harriet LaBarre's *Plastic Surgery: Beauty You Can Buy* and *Dr. Make Me Beautiful,* by James W. Smith and Samm S. Baker, are good, readable surveys of what can be done. Other books are available at your bookstore or library. Your family physician may be able to recommend a surgeon. If not, your local medical society can help.

As a final word on the subject of cosmetic surgery, let me offer an opinion rather than more facts. The cosmetic surgeon's goal is to make his patient more attractive. Successful surgery improves the appearance, but I believe that its greatest value is not the "artistic" or physical change, but the new confidence that so often accompanies such procedures.

Lawrence, a forty-five-year-old writer whom I treated, illustrates this well. He had always taken care of his physical health, and was one of those fortunate individuals who was able to "shake off" the few colds, bouts of bursitis, and minor infections that he encountered with a minimum of complications. I had always envied his stamina, necessary in his work as a free-lance journalist who did a great deal of traveling. But one day as we went over his test results, all of which were good, I could sense he had a problem.

"Congratulations," I said. "If all my patients were as healthy as you are, I'd be able to cut down my office hours."

Lawrence always had an excellent sense of humor, but his smile was halfhearted.

"Maybe I'm in good health," he said, "but I wish I looked better."

I'd examined him thoroughly, and he looked fine to me. But so often, I've discovered, a patient can tell more about his problems than a doctor can discover in the examining room. "Do you think you don't look well?" I asked.

Lawrence shrugged his shoulders. "Oh, it's not that I look sick. But doctor, it seems as though all the magazines are hiring young editors. Even the people who make news these days—the politicians, the executives, and the various people I write about—are so young. I feel as though they think of me as an old man."

I gave his face a close look, and he removed the lightly tinted sunglasses he'd been wearing. His eyes, I noticed, were surrounded by a web of fine lines, and there were slightly discolored swellings beneath them. It wasn't unnatural or unbecoming, but it was disturbing to Lawrence, and that was what mattered.

"You know," he said, "lately I've missed a few good assignments I've gone after. Not because of my writing, either, but because I didn't come across as young enough. My field is very competitive, and though experience counts, I just can't help wishing I didn't look forty-five— even if it's a healthy forty-five."

I'd heard similar complaints many times before from male patients. Often I had to probe and prod to find the root of the problem, working my way through several layers of misconceptions—primarily that there is something unmasculine about being concerned with one's appearance. The growth of the male cosmetic industry belies this sexist attitude. I was glad that Lawrence had been so direct: I could be direct too.

"If it really bothers you," I told him, "why not have some cosmetic surgery done?"

"Me? Have a face lift?" he asked, surprised but not rejecting the idea, either.

I told him that I wasn't suggesting a full face lift, or any particular procedure, for that matter. But there were, I explained, a number of possibilities that he could explore, and in his specific case, an "eye lift" seemed worth investigating.

"The main thing I'm saying," I told him, "is that you can do something about your appearance besides worry about it. I've seen a number of men your age—some of them executives who had to find new jobs and felt very self-conscious about looking older than the competition—have cosmetic surgery with excellent results."

He said he'd think it over, and asked for the name of a cosmetic surgeon "just in case" he decided to pursue the subject further. That was the last I heard until a month later, when he showed up in my office without his sunglasses.

"Well?" he asked.

"Well what?" I answered. "I'm going to have to ask you what's wrong. You certainly don't look sick to me."

"Come on, Dr. Parrish. Don't you notice the difference?"

I studied his face, and saw that the bags under his eyes were gone. He'd had the operation, and he'd even managed to turn the experience into a magazine article.

"I feel as though I'm a new man," he said. "I like the way I look. Don't you think it's a big improvement?"

I had to agree that it was, though not entirely for the same reasons as Lawrence. From a purely physical standpoint, his face was probably more attractive. The bags under his eyes were gone, and the lines were fewer. The big change, though, was in his attitude. He felt better about himself, more confident and less self-conscious. I had a feeling that he'd get the assignments he had missed, but that it wouldn't be the new look to his face that would be responsible as much as his attitude.

For men as well as women, self-image is terribly important. How we see ourselves dictates, to a large extent, how others see us. Cosmetic surgery and related procedures can make a physical change, but they can also afford psychological benefits. The confidence and satisfaction an individual can take in believing he looks well is as important as any change a surgeon makes in the actual appearance.

When a man or woman is unhappy with the way he or she looks, other people sense it. It isn't always a matter of verbalizing complaints, though some people do that, too, but it's a matter of carriage and interaction with others. The woman who can walk into a room with her head high and a warm confident smile on her face is automatically attractive—whether she is sixteen or sixty, and whether she's had cosmetic surgery or not.

For some people, this particular attitude is instinctive, or ingrained from childhood. Sometimes I've found that the most attractive women at a party or a dinner aren't the ones with the perfect features; often they're obsessed with what time is doing to their natural assets, and the obsession shows in the constant search for "just the right light" or the tilt of a head designed to show her best angle but showing, instead, a wooden rigidity.

Yet there are those women who, particularly at the time of the climacteric, feel a kind of panic about their appearance. It may not be just a matter of lines and wrinkles, but of the total body. They realize they are getting older, and that the aging process is showing. Often the reaction is to set out in search of a miracle of some sort, like Rosalyn, the wife of a successful banker.

Neither Rosalyn nor her husband were patients of mine, but we had seen each other socially at the homes of mutual friends on a number of occasions. One night, after a dinner, the subject of beauty spas came up, and I listened with interest as various women recounted their experiences at The Golden Door, Main Chance, and La Costa.

Later, over coffee, Rosalyn sat beside me in our hostess' living room.

"I think I'm going to go to a spa for a couple of weeks. Tell me, since you're a doctor, do you think it's a good idea?"

"Why not go?" I suggested. "You can afford it."

She looked at me with her eyes wide. "But surely that isn't the main reason. . . ."

I told her that it most decidedly was. Mud packs, masks, massages aside, the primary thing that beauty spas offer is a chance to be pampered, and there is hardly a woman—or a man, for that matter—who will not prosper in such an atmosphere. Unfortunately, beauty spas are expensive and few of us can afford them.

The woman who feels that she "just has to do something" about the way she looks can be lured by brochures that promise "two weeks can change your whole life," and she may believe that nothing short of hopping a jet for the spa promising the most will help her.

Spas can be helpful for the atmosphere of indulgence they offer, but as far as "miracles" go, much of the supposedly miraculous is in the mind of the believer. And much of what is accomplished at a beauty spa can be accomplished at home.

Sophie Green was a woman who wanted a miracle. She was one of the first private patients I treated. Over the years I had seen her through bronchitis, gastritis, bursitis, and vaginitis, among other problems, and most recently I'd seen her through a menopausal syndrome, which became critical on the death of her husband.

If anyone had called Sophie pretty, she'd probably have laughed in his face. If somebody had called her a great party girl, however, she'd have agreed at once. She played the piano, relished the latest gossip (of which she had an endless supply), and kept up Scotch for Scotch with the drinkers at any party she attended. She was very much a life-of-the-party type, and as a result, invitations flew her way in great quantity.

When her husband died, however, things changed. For months Sophie didn't go out, but busied herself cooking and eating. When, at last, she began to accept invitations, she inevitably came home early—in time for a midnight snack that often meant another meal even bigger than the dinner her host or hostess had provided.

Her depression wasn't severe, but she needed supportive therapy. She needed to talk, and I was glad to listen. I had always enjoyed our easy relationship, and over the time I saw her on a regular basis, a mutual fondness had developed. During those first months following the death of her husband, I tried to help Sophie understand her feelings. She'd gone through a tragedy, and depression was a natural reaction to the loss she felt.

We spoke about her feelings in our weekly sessions, and I monitored her physical health, cautioning her about her eating, which was becoming a serious problem. But I felt that her main need was support and tenderness. A turning point would come in time.

It came shortly after Sophie decided to go back to work. She took a job with a law firm, and in the following weeks she met a partner, a widower who was readjusting to living alone. He was looking for someone to party with, Sophie informed me, and they'd gone out together several times. Over the next few months the relationship continued to blossom—but so did Sophie's weight.

She'd tried diet after diet, she insisted, whenever we talked about what was now an obesity problem, but "something was wrong." She refused to believe that the problem wasn't the diet, but rather her failure to stick to it. She had read about a spa that promised to "melt the pounds off," and she'd arranged to take two weeks off and go.

"Just look at this!" Sophie proclaimed, reaching into her tote bag for a copy of one of the fashion magazines. She flashed a picture at me, and I recognized the model as an actress in a television series. "She just raves about the place, and look at what it's done for her."

"I don't think that girl weighed in at the spa at 177 pounds," I said, as gently as possible. "Do you?"

Sophie's face dropped. "But I have to do something. And at a spa, they'll do it for me."

Sophie had put into words the feeling that so many women have: spas, somehow, do the work. The pounds roll off and the years fly backward through magic. It simply is not the case.

Sophie, I decided, had been coddled enough. It was time for some hard facts.

"If you want to go to the spa, have a good time," I said. "But go as a realist, please, for your own sake. What the spa will do is put you on a strict diet, which isn't exactly an idea you haven't heard before, and encourage you to do some exercise—which I seem to remember mentioning a dozen or so times. There are no miracles, and nobody is going to do anything about your weight and figure problems except you."

Sophie went to her spa, but two weeks after her return she was back in my office. She had managed to lose a few pounds, but the minute she left the spa, she had reverted to her old eating habits, and now she was right back where she had started. But she had learned something: spas could take off weight, but only willpower could keep it off. She asked me to prescribe a diet, and this time she seemed resolved to stick to it.

Sophie kept her word. It was not easy, but she was highly motivated and her new gentleman friend helped to pull her back when she found herself slipping. It took several months, but she lost the weight. A year later Sophie was a new woman—with a new morale to match.

Appearance can be the main motivation for a weight control program, but from a medical point of view, weight control is an essential part of good health, and it is particularly important in the middle years. As the metabolism slows, the body puts on weight more easily—too easily, for most people. The rate of activity isn't the only thing that slows down: life-styles become more sedentary.

It is essential to take a commonsense approach to the foods we eat, not only in order to look better, but to live longer, healthier lives. One positive change in our society is a growing awareness of nutrition. We've moved away from the time when we ate without thinking about anything more than taste. Today we are aware (or should be) of calories, carbohydrates, fats, protein, sodium, and the fatty acid content of foods.

A few commonsense facts can be very helpful, and certainly common sense should go hand in hand with any diet, along with an examination by a physician. Fad diets, so popular these days, are an extension of the same attitude my patient Sophie had about the beauty spa—the idea that a miraculous change could somehow occur. I don't condemn fad dieting, though I don't recommend it, either. A few days of a fad diet can lead to an initial weight loss that can motivate the man or woman who wants to reduce. For some, however, the imbalance of nutrients in many of these diets outweighs any possible benefits; a key reason why your doctor should be consulted before you start.

At best, fad diets are designed to be used for short

periods of time. Ultimately, we must change our eating habits if we are to maintain a healthy weight. But a change in eating habits is important in other aspects of health as well.

A good beginning is breaking the American habit of oversalting our food, and thereby reducing our sodium intake. Sodium gets into the cells and, through the process of osmosis, causes them to retain water. This not only increases the body's weight, but also the workload on the heart. Slowly cut down on the amount of salt you use in cooking and the amount you add at the table. Everyone should break the habit of salting food before he tastes it. Gourmets and doctors, on this point at least, are in total agreement.

In addition to avoiding sodium, the intake of fatty acids, saturated and unsaturated, should be examined. Both are high in calories, and saturated fatty acids (animal fats) are high in cholesterol and triglycerides, which contribute to hardening of the arteries. These substances are deposited in the arteries, including those in the wall of the heart and in the heart valves. They become calcified, and the arteries lose their elasticity and strength. These calcifications or plaques narrow the vessels, impair the flow of blood, elevate the blood pressure, and promote clots or thromboses. These factors combined are the basic cause of heart attacks and strokes.

Avoiding animal fats and fatty dairy products is a good idea at any age, but it is particularly important as we get older. Red meats, even when trimmed (do your trimming before you cook them, getting rid of as much fat as you can) are high in saturated fats. If frying meat is a habit, break it. Instead, broil your meats, or if you are roasting them, use a rack in your baking pan so the meat doesn't sit in the fat you're trying to cook out.

Sensible eating, both for weight loss and for general

good health, may sound like a deprivation. It isn't; it's a challenge. Instead of a well-marbled steak, use your creativity with a leaner cut of meat. The marbling that we equate with prime meat is, keep in mind, fat.

Learn to balance your sources of protein. Fish (shellfish is the exception in cholesterol terms) and chicken are good protein sources, as are soy beans and skimmed milk.

Almost every day, it seems, brings news about the reported benefit or harm of some food or food group. Knowing what to eat can be confusing, but the confusion lessens if you try to remember that a diet balanced in variety is the most healthful. Moderation in terms of the type of food you eat—and the amount—is a good guideline.

Your doctor can advise you on foods to either eat or avoid depending on your own health problems. Some people have a high level of uric acid in their blood, and this can cause gouty arthritis and is probably another predisposing factor to diseases of the circulatory system. Animal organs, beans, sardines, anchovies, mushrooms, and meat extracts are to be avoided in cases where uric acid is a problem.

If water retention is a problem, not only should salt be avoided, but also foods that have a naturally high sodium content.

As we get older, many of us have bowel problems. Roughage is good. It promotes regularity and guards against cancer of the colon. And be sure to eat fresh food whenever possible. The fresher the food, the higher the vitamin and mineral content. That is not to say that canned and frozen vegetables are lacking in vitamins, but just as there is more nutritive content in a tomato that comes from your garden than in one that's spent several days on the supermarket shelf, there's more in a fresh tomato than one that comes from a can.

Fortunately, food manufacturers have come a long way in terms of making a wide variety of foods for special diets. They do the best they can to make their products palatable, and some of the results are very good. In shopping for food, though, be sure to study labels carefully. "Diet" means a prescribed eating program, and what's good for weight loss may not be good for a special problem, and vice versa.

An excess of carbohydrates isn't good for anyone's weight or health, though some carbohydrates are needed for the metabolism. Avoid, whenever possible, white sugar and bleached flour. Recognize, too, that there is a link between the mind and body. Coffee contains caffeine, as do certain soft drinks, particularly colas. Since caffeine is a stimulant, these anxiety-promoting beverages are to be avoided when you are feeling nervous or before bedtime.

A healthy diet doesn't have to taste bad; it just demands a bit of discretion. Low-calorie foods and sugar and salt substitutes can frequently be used without radically altering the taste of a favorite dish. And if you watch your diet, as a general rule you can afford a moderate portion of a particularly high-calorie favorite from time to time, unless your doctor advises otherwise.

Obesity is not only unattractive, is is downright dangerous. It contributes to hypertension, heart disease, and diabetes. When these problems occur, obesity increases the severity. Should a surgical problem come up, obesity makes surgery of any sort more dangerous.

And, too, it has a kind of self-promoting effect. The individual who is overweight doesn't like the way he looks. Movement, if he or she is obese, can be difficult or even painful. Many an overweight patient of mine has admitted that it's a lot easier to sit home eating pie a la mode than it is to exercise, and activity is essential at this time of life.

Nobody can argue with the cosmetic benefits on this subject: exercise does, most definitely, help firm up muscles. But beware of the tendency to overdo, or to do too much too fast.

Every community has more than its share of "reducing salons," and while some are staffed with competent professionals, many are professional only in terms of high-pressure salesmanship. These people know that most of us find exercising at home alone, boring. Salons offer an atmosphere of conviviality and luxury, but too often they offer little or no proper supervision or guidance.

Keeping physically active is good for slimming down and toning muscles, as well as maintaining their strength. The bones, too, need stress to promote normal metabolism and to retard demineralization. Lazy joints—with or without the presence of an arthritic condition—tend to become stiff. "Grease" them with activity, be it walking, dancing, or knitting.

It is never too late to start living healthier, or to get interested in a sport or activity. If you want to meet people, take up tennis or swimming. Dancing—ballroom or square dancing—gets you into an entertaining social situation as well as into action. Or exercise can be simple: why not get the bridge club to go for a nice long hike? Gossip is just as much fun on the move as it is over the card table.

When we think of exercise, we think of movement, but too often we forget basic, daily activity. It's exercising when you walk the few blocks to the store instead of taking the bus. Sitting, standing, and walking erect not only help you to present a more attractive figure in terms of posture, but help to shape up the muscles, especially those of the abdomen. Good posture keeps the spine in the proper position. It also positions the thorax for maximum expansion of all the lung tissue and inflation of the most peripheral lung sacs for optimal oxygen-carbon dioxide exchange. In other words, it not only helps you look better, but makes you feel better.

Very often, the man or woman who has had a physical injury, or an illness, or a coronary is afraid of exercise. Caution is common sense, and in cases of this type it's always essential to ask your doctor how much you can and should do. But exercise and activity, particularly after illness, help us to get reinvolved with life, and prevent invalidism. Patients benefit from becoming more secure in their ability to be active. If a recent illness or health problem makes you afraid of activity, be sure to bring this problem to your doctor. He'll understand, and he may recommend a physical rehabilitation program perfectly suited to your needs.

Whether you are exercising for good health or for weight loss, keep one rule in mind: activity should produce *healthy* stress, not exhaustion. The crash-diet syndrome is closely linked to the overdo-exercise pattern. Too many patients who should have known better, and doubtless would have if they'd let common sense rather than vanity dictate, have come to my office literally aching all over from a one-day spurt of excessive exercise.

You can best judge how much exercise you can handle. If you've read something in a book or magazine, an exercise to firm the abdomen, and the instructions say to repeat the exercise five times, that doesn't mean your efforts will be fruitless if you can only do the exercise twice without discomfort. There is a thin line between stress and strain, between pushing our bodies toward the limit and beyond it.

Try to do some exercise every day, even if it's just a walk around the block. Recently a patient of mine told me about his mother.

"She has arthritis and is in constant pain," he said, "but

each morning she turns on the television and watches an exercise program. Getting out of bed is painful after a night's sleep, so she does what exercises she can do in bed. Jack LaLanne may be doing jumping jacks, but my mother moves her arms up and down. The movement, she says, gets her started—and makes getting out of bed easier."

It's a commendable effort, and an excellent example of using inventiveness in a personalized exercise program.

Remember, too, that certain times of the day are better for exercising than others. Avoid physical activity immediately after eating, and also before retiring, when increased circulation can make it difficult to fall asleep.

Two weeks at a beauty spa? If you can afford the time and the money, fine. It's delightful to have someone else cooking slimming, healthful meals and leading you through an exercise program. But even those who are lucky enough to go to beauty spas must come back to reality—and the reality is that healthful eating and regular activity are important to looking and feeling our best every day of our lives.

Sex After Forty

Sexual Activity During the Climacteric

"You've made me feel a lot better, Dr. Parrish," Helene, my patient, said as our appointment came to an end. "I suppose it sounds silly, but I was actually afraid of the climacteric."

"There's nothing to worry about," I assured her. "You've taken good care of yourself. Watching your diet the way you've done really pays dividends. Your cholesterol level is excellent, and both you and Charles have had regular checkups. If you'll just take the estrogen supplement I prescribed, I think that you and your husband can look forward to a lot of happy years together."

Helene smiled, but a rather wistful expression caught my attention. "You're not upset about something, are you?" I asked.

"Dr. Parrish, I keep forgetting that you are a psychiatrist as well as a GP," Helene answered. "It's the reaction of a silly lady, I guess. I should be very happy with what you've told me, and I am. But I'm thinking of what you said about Charles and me. We probably do have a lot of years left together, but I guess we're going to have to start living more as friends than lovers. It's going to be quite an adjustment."

I felt that I'd missed something, and I asked Helene to explain.

"Oh, you know what I'm talking about," my patient said. "The climacteric, the middle-age crisis, menopause—whatever you want to call it, it means the end of a sex life. I know that."

Once the dam was broken, Helene's feelings and fears began to pour out. Her husband, she believed, was losing interest in her as a woman. Though he was still considerate and attentive, she was convinced that he had lost his sexual desire for her. Her own sex drive, she confided, had also tapered off. Even when she and Charles had sexual relations, she told me, she found them much less satisfying than they had been earlier in the marriage, and often she had trouble reaching a climax.

When she finished, Helene was trying to keep a firm hold on her emotions, and making an equally determined effort to blame herself for bringing up the subject in the first place.

"Just forget my ramblings," she urged me. "Lots of women my age have serious medical problems. I should be grateful that I'm as well off as I am. As for sex—well, I'll just have to get used to living without it."

"But why?" I asked. "There's no reason whatsoever why you and Charles can't enjoy a full and active sex life, not only now, but for many years to come. Everything changes with time, sex included. But at this point in your life, your sexual relationship with your husband could change for the better, if you'd change some of your thinking."

She stared at me in amazement, but listened attentively

as I began to discuss the neglected subject of sex and the climacteric.

Over the years, there have been many women like Helene in my office, and a comparable number of male counterparts. The myth that an individual's sex life fades away or ends when he reaches a certain time of life is so widespread that it crosses lines of gender, education, and sophistication. Women frequently tell me, with little concern for hard evidence, that they've lost their desirability. Their husbands, they complain, have begun calling them—and treating them like—Mother. Or single women suddenly complain that men look at them only as potential friends, rather than complete females. Another frequent complaint is that when sexual relations take place, it is no longer enjoyable. Some women say the experience leaves them feeling "empty." Others complain of physical discomfort and pain.

Men, too, have a wide variety of problems. They're afraid that sexual potency is something that vanishes with the vigor of youth. Such negative attitudes detract from their sexuality and—like self-fulfilling prophecies— impair their performance. As a result, they present me with problems of damaged egos and real or imagined inability to satisfy themselves or their partner.

All of these complaints can be legitimate, but the causes are far more specific than the commonly accepted ideas of being "too far along in years" to enjoy sex. And like most legitimate mental and physical complaints, these specific problems can be treated with counseling, supportive therapy, and medical help. Certainly nothing is to be gained—and half a lifetime to be lost—by giving up.

Sex, quite simply, does *not* end at some prescribed point in the life cycle, the climacteric notwithstanding. In spite of all the proverbial old wives' tales, the climacteric and postclimacteric years can and should be rich and sexually satisfying.

The greatest hindrance to this goal is not basically a medical problem, but rather a common misconception which, after years of social conditioning, has translated itself into a psychological fact for many people. If you believe that your sexual existence will change drastically or come to an end at a given time in life, it's very likely that it will. Sex, after all, is a state of mind as much as body.

The roots of this particular sexual myth are probably founded, oddly enough, in physiological fact. The cessation of the menses marks the end of a woman's capacity to reproduce. Within the context of their view that sex was "good" only in its reproductive function, our Victorian forebears were only too happy to interpret the physical menopause as a sign that a woman's "obligation" to her husband was over.

The Victorian ethic directly influenced many of us, particularly when it met up with the puritan tradition on American shores. As a result, many of those experiencing or about to experience the climacteric may be influenced by these attitudes, and their first step toward establishing a healthy and happy sex life may be a deconditioning.

More recent generations, particularly those growing up in the age of the "new morality," will not have this problem. Changes in morality and mores are, of course, matters of personal decision, and one need not accept or approve all of them to enjoy a happy sex life.

Like my patient Helene, many women feel that the physical menopause signals a cessation of their sexual attraction. The monthly reaffirmation of their femininity has stopped, they reason; therefore, they are sexless. This deduction, quite obviously, is not the result of a logical process, but the expression of a fear.

"My insides are drying up," more than one patient has told me, often in tears. Women who view the menopause this way often feel that their sexual desire and their desirability are "drying up" as well.

We can look forward to a decline in this problem in coming years as our social attitudes toward the menstrual cycle continue to change. The widespread use of oral contraceptives among women can produce monthly bleeding after the natural function of the ovaries has declined. A few women can continue to take "the pill" for a time after it is needed, for the psychological benefit of an artificial menstrual period. Their femininity is reinforced by the continuation of the biological function which they associate with being a woman.

The woman who is taking oral contraceptives as she enters the climacteric is confronted with an obvious question: if birth control pills produce monthly bleeding, how does she know if her natural menses have ceased? In some cases, the best way to make this determination is through the simple test of stopping birth control pills to see if menstruation still occurs. This, however—and it should be stressed—is not a do-it-yourself project. Most doctors would prefer that patients presented them with this question.

An examination and some testing may quickly determine whether or not a patient has entered the menopause. At the very least, a physician can advise a safe alternate form of birth control to be used while the determination is being made. Late pregnancies, though infrequent, can and do happen.

A forty-eight-year-old patient of mine decided that it was time for her to go off oral contraceptives to see if she had entered the menopause. She attributed her bleeding, a few weeks after she stopped taking the medication, to an aftereffect, and the following month, when the days she'd marked on her calendar came and went with no sign of a menstrual period, she announced to her friends that menopause had occurred. A few weeks later she phoned with complaints of weakness and nausea. Tests proved, to her surprise, that she was pregnant, though complications prevented her from carrying the pregnancy to term. A great deal of unhappiness might have been avoided had she checked with me before stopping the birth control pills, or if she and her husband had had the foresight to use an alternate form of birth control.

The pill contains estrogen, and in many women the amount of estrogen it contains, when added to the gradually declining supply produced by the ovaries, can delay the physical symptoms of the climacteric. That does not mean, as some believe, that taking oral contraceptives can permanently forestall the menopause or menopausal symptoms. That is not their purpose.

Physical symptoms aside, the fact is that the decline of a woman's hormone supply has *no direct effect* on a woman's sexuality. She is not like other animals with menstrual cycles whose sexual response is controlled by hormones. Women do not go into—or out of—"heat." Countless studies have failed to demonstrate any link between her hormones and sexual desire or capability. The cessation of the menses is absolutely unconnected with sexual activity.

Of course, physical and emotional problems that result from estrogen deficiency can indirectly affect sexual desire and response.

Of sexual difficulties, the most common physical complaint expressed by women during the climacteric is that of painful intercourse. Often this problem is compounded by the lack of understanding shown by sex partners. Even a devoted husband may find it hard to understand why, after years or decades of marriage, his wife suddenly finds sexual relations painful and unpleasant. He may interpret this complaint as a rejection.

Pain during intercourse is a very real and legitimate complaint. As we have seen, a decline of natural estrogen can produce an atrophy, or shrinking, of vaginal tissue. In addition, the cells of the vaginal tissue slow down and no longer furnish their natural lubricants. As a result, the vagina may become tender—in some cases, raw. Intercourse is naturally painful and irritating.

This atrophic vaginitis, however, is very easily treated. ERT has a speedy and positive effect. Topical estrogen creams alone may provide relief. Every case must, of course, be treated individually, but your doctor may prescribe the use of a topical cream containing estrogen and soothing agents for local relief, along with an oral estrogen supplement that will help correct this and other problems.

As the natural pH, or acid/alkali balance of the vagina changes, other problems present themselves. Infection, such as an overgrowth of yeast, can also make sexual relations—not only intercourse, but touching or any form of foreplay—painful. But these complaints, too, are treatable.

It is much more dangerous, in terms of a marriage or sexual relationship as well as the patient's well-being, to let these problems go unchecked. Let's suppose, for example, that a woman begins to experience vaginal atrophy. Intercourse begins to become painful, rather than pleasurable. She shies away from it, or submits reluctantly out of a desire to please her husband—or, often, out of a fear of rejecting him.

She may decline to discuss the problem with her husband, feeling that it is too intimate or too personal. If she tries to discuss it with him, he may not understand. At the same time, however, many women are hesitant to bring such problems to their family doctor, either out of embarrassment or fear that the symptoms are signs of some grave problem.

The vast majority of such complaints are common and easily treatable. Doctors are familiar with them, and treatment and relief are readily available. In short, it is much more simple to treat these complaints than it is to repair the breakdown of communications in a marriage that they can lead to—or the fear of sex that can overcome a woman if these problems go unchecked.

Medical problems are often compounded by home remedy approaches, and vaginal irritations are no exception. In recent years, Madison Avenue has discovered feminine hygiene. A multitude of new products, and a battery of advertisements promoting their uses, are conditioning women to douche excessively.

In the absence of disease, the effect of douching is more psychologically than physically or hygienically beneficial. In fact, excessive douching, particularly with strong preparations, can be dangerous. The vagina harbors bacteria that guard against infection. If these are destroyed by strong chemicals, discomfort or disease can result. Certainly this is a liability in estrogen-deficient women where the normal acid-alkali balance is already upset. Overgrowth of naturally occurring yeast can cause vaginal problems.

If a woman feels the need to douche, an excellent preparation can be made by mixing a tablespoon of vinegar with a quart of warm water. This may even help maintain the necessary acidity. Normal bathing insures cleanliness for most women, but if you feel that frequent douching is essential, you should check the douche you use with your doctor.

In the absence of physical symptoms, it's likely that a decline in sexual responsiveness is a repercussion of emotional problems. The mood swings, depressions, and tensions associated with this period of life contribute to a variety of sexual problems. Even with all other factors positive, the psychological state naturally engendered by the climacteric hardly creates a mood of romance. A woman who feels that she is losing her attractiveness, that she is no longer pleasant to look at or desirable as a woman, may view sex as a test—one she may refuse to take for fear she won't pass.

The climacteric's emotional aspects also tend to make many people introverted. Simple conversation and the everyday emotions of interpersonal relationships can become an ordeal. A patient whose marriage problems brought her to me for treatment during the climacteric summed up the chain reaction that can occur.

"I've gotten so that I can't talk to anyone," she confided. "And Doctor Parrish, I *like* people! For years I've played cards every week with the same group of women. Now, losing a hand or some innocent remark one of my friends makes can actually start me crying. It's the same with my husband. He hasn't done anything at all, I find when I really think about it, but almost every time we talk I get upset or burst into tears. In the past few months, I've practically become a recluse. I'm just not fit to be with other people—including my husband!"

This patient's insight into her own behavior was the key to solving her problems—which she did with a little counseling and therapy.

Self-analysis is a good starting place toward solving sexual problems. When a woman comes to me complaining that she's lost her desire for her husband, I try not to counsel so much as to listen, prodding with questions. What does she really feel she's lost? What is really upsetting her? Once her thinking is directed along these lines, a woman can often find the answers in herself.

It would be wrong to imply that sexual problems during the middle years all revolve around the female partner. Like women, men have specific difficulties, and on the whole men are much more reluctant to discuss them.

Paramount among the real and psychosomatic problems that the middle-aged man is confronted with is impotence—or, more properly, "functional impotence": the inability to achieve and maintain an erection. Although sexual stereotypes are changing as a result of social awareness, for many men, the penis is still the measure of masculinity. A continuing functional impotence can destroy a man's self-image, as well as his marriage.

Many such men turn to their physician with requests for "miracle" hormones. The fact is, that a hormone deficiency is not the usual cause of reduced sexual response or impotence. Even so, hormone injections can sometimes produce a psychological response that can ease a temporary physical problem. I have a patient, a stockbroker, whose erections seem to be a direct reflection of the stock market. When he comes in and asks for a hormone shot, I know the market is down. I recall another patient who made a convenient marriage with a rich and socially prominent woman who loved to travel. Their relationship had never been—in any way—a very good one, but for the sake of their children they had stayed together. During her seasons in the Caribbean or on the Riviera I never saw him. But I always knew when she had returned to the city; he would be in twice a week for his injections.

From a scientific standpoint, I don't think that in either of these cases the amount of testosterone received increased potency. But what mattered was that they thought it did. I find that often a mild tranquilizer is just as effective. By relieving some of the anxiety that perpetuates a patient's impotency, his response can improve markedly. And a single success can start a new, positive cycle that will reinforce that success.

Otherwise, an initial failure to reach or sustain an erection may lead a man into a trap of self-doubt and depression. His masculinity, he may decide, is gone—along with his youth. His sexual problem can begin to color his entire life, affecting his relationships, his home life, and his work.

Depression, a frequent factor in impotency, is a two-edged sword. Not only does the fear of impotence produce depression, but depression itself, not uncommon at this time of life, contributes to impotence.

Men and women, it must be remembered, differ in their psychological attitude toward sex. While each of us, male and female, has his or her own, very personal view of sex, women on the whole tend to romanticize the subject more than men. Men are likely to retain more of their adolescent, "proving ground" associations.

The man who is confronted with the fact that he is middle-aged, that he is no longer a "young man on the way up" but a mature male who has completed the broad outlines of his life, may be depressed by his failure to have accomplished all he set out to. His youth and his chance, he may feel, are but a memory. In this depressed state, temporary impotence reflects his sense of loss.

The acceptance of oneself and the inevitable process of time, is often the best treatment for this type of sexual problem. This is the approach I try to use with male patients who come to me for help, but frequently a man will look for answers in other places—including extramarital sex.

It is easier for all of us, men and women alike, to blame others for our problems than it is to examine ourselves. The man who has encountered a sexual dysfunction such as impotence may place the blame on his wife. He can come up with a variety of rationalizations: his mate is unresponsive; after a number of years of marriage, the excitement of sex has dissipated; he will stray from fidelity just once, or just long enough to "prove" himself.

It is possible that another woman will provide an atmosphere free of tensions associated with marriage and, in a broader sense, his real life, that will enable him to perform sexually. It is also quite likely, particularly if he has been a faithful, devoted husband previously, that he will feel guilty, thereby defeating the purpose of the extramarital tryst on an immediate basis and, in the long term, adding to his self-recrimination and depression.

When men finally do discuss impotence with their doctors, they usually come in totally dejected and frightened that the end has begun, that some dread disease has begun.

There are relatively few cases where physiological or neurological factors cause impotence, and I am quick to point this out to patients, to their great relief. True hormone deficiency, as I have noted, is usually not the cause. Other factors that might possibly play a part include injuries to the spinal cord or brain, undiagnosed diabetes, hepatic problems, and prostatic conditions. Any or all of these can affect the libido, and the physical ability to achieve an erection. These factors, however, are far less common than stress, fatigue, and depression.

I also ask patients to list any and all medications they may be taking. Certain drugs, particularly those used for hypertension, mood elevation, and anxiety, can have side effects that inhibit erection and ejaculation, as can abuse of narcotics and alcohol.

A change of medication may be indicated, but in most cases the treatment of impotence is based on psychological counseling. This is not to say that when a man finds himself unable to get an erection, the problem is imaginary. But, as I remind all my patients with such complaints, the ability to gain an erection at any time— waking with a "morning erection" or an occasional arousal during the day—effectively rules out true physical impotence.

It should be remembered that the sex drive of every person is not the same. Not only does it vary from individual to individual, but it can vary during different periods of one's life. As metabolism slows, various drives and energies slow, sex included. It is not physically necessary, in most men, to ejaculate as frequently as it once was. The man who tries, at forty-five, to equal the sexual frequency he had at age twenty, may be making excessive demands on his body.

Legitimate psychological factors and those that have no substantive foundation must be separated. Not long ago, a patient of mine came in with a complaint that had absolutely no validity. Knowing that Henry was a teacher, and a well-read man, I must admit that it took me by surprise.

"I think I have what's commonly called a case for the books," he informed me. "I don't suppose that you'll believe me, Dr. Parrish, but my penis is shrinking!"

Henry believed this sincerely, and told me that the reflection of his nude image in the mirror proved he was right. I quickly checked his chart, noting that he had gained twenty pounds in the past few years. His increased girth and the buildup of fat in the lower abdominal and groin areas seemed to have made his penis look smaller. When I pointed this out, Henry was relieved—and his relief made it easier to treat his second complaint, impotence.

The male genitalia does not "shrivel up" or diminish in size with age. In the postclimacteric years the female genitalia can atrophy with hormonal deprivation, and this is often accompanied by a loss of pubic hair. To many women, this loss of prominent external genitalia can be very depressing and inhibiting to their sexuality. Fortunately, the atrophy can be partially corrected with estrogen replacement.

Most of us, when we see our reflection, don't react as extremely as my patient Henry, but what we see and how we react to it can greatly affect our sexual responsiveness. The man or woman who measures the reality of his appearance at the time of the climacteric against a remembered picture of what he or she looked like a quarter of a century before, is doomed to be disappointed. All of us grow older—and learning to accept that fact is a mark of the maturing process, a process as continual as life itself.

That does not mean that we must accept what we see as what we must be. People in the middle years have a great capacity to improve their appearance, and the effort to do so pays great psychological as well as aesthetic dividends. The man who sets out to lose twenty extra pounds that he has gradually accumulated—a patient like Henry, for example—not only looks better, but feels better as a result of having done something for himself and asserted his will. The woman who decides to exercise sensibly and tone up her body will like herself better and better as she begins to achieve her goal.

Feeling that you are desirable makes you desirable, and promotes a more satisfying sexual existence.

Unfortunately, instead of looking to ourselves, we often search for outside sources of stimulation. Since the dawn of time, people have sought the magic potion of aphrodisia. But no such potion has been found—and, I must add, I do not think one ever will. People should turn to themselves and to each other to find the secret formula. Sex and sexual arousal is ideally linked to love. When we speak of self-image, we should not neglect the self-image that comes of seeing oneself in the eyes of a life partner.

It is not uncommon for a husband and wife to be going through the climacteric at approximately the same time. Such a situation, needless to say, can be very complex. A man may look at his wife as she goes through the symptoms of the menopause and realize that he, too, is getting older. He may sympathize, but may be too deeply immersed in his own depression to offer the patience and support that she needs. This situation works both ways: a woman may know that her husband is depressed, under stress, and going through a difficult time of life, but her own symptoms may be too overwhelming for her to comfort him.

The middle-age crisis can draw people closer together, or push them apart. The choice depends, to a large extent, on communication.

"But I *know* Harry," a patient will insist when I mention this.

"Come on, Doc—I've been married to Marge for twenty-five years" a man will say.

I gently point out that time, in a marriage, is not an insurance policy. It can work the other way, in truth, creating a situation in which husband and wife take each other for granted. So many little things go unspoken that big things—feelings, fears, and emotions—often go unexpressed as well.

Counseling can help. And contrary to popular opinion, that doesn't mean that a couple need be in serious trouble or need embark on an extensive therapy program to benefit from it. In one or two sessions, a doctor can outline the climacteric, along with how husband and wife can help each other. Given the opportunity, I've found in numerous cases, husband and wife will share feelings that aren't expressed over the dinner table or during television commercials.

During such sessions, I urge patients to focus on what *is* rather than what *was*, and I believe that this viewpoint can make for a better sex life. By the time a man or woman reaches the climacteric, children, in all likelihood, have left home to marry or start careers. Much as parents love their children, having them in the house can be an inhibiting factor in sexual relations. The middle years bring a special freedom, sometimes the very first chance in years to enjoy romance.

As I tell my patients, it is very difficult to enjoy a quiet, leisurely meal, complete with candlelight, soft music, and a bottle of wine, when little Johnny and his sister are fighting at the table. Romance is one of the world's greatest luxuries, and the middle years are the years when it can be best indulged, enjoyed and appreciated.

We often go to great effort, men and women alike, to dress attractively and make ourselves look our best to go out, if only to a dinner with friends or to a movie. Naturally, at these times husband and wife are proud of each other's appearance, but making that extra bit of effort to look as attractive as you can for your mate, for a romantic dinner or a quiet evening at home, is a kind of gift. It shows that you care. It is appreciated. And it is returned.

The middle years, then, can be a time for rediscovery. Vacations are an ideal way of perking up a sex life—and a marriage in general. A few weeks or even days away from the normal stresses and responsibilities of daily life can give you the time to fully enjoy each other.

Sex at this time of life can also be a source of discovery. Just as many aspects of a relationship can be taken for granted over a number of years, sex can become routine. Making love the exact same way year after year undoubtedly induces a kind of monotony. Varying the type of sexual activity helps greatly.

"But how do I start?" a patient of mine asked when I gave him this advice. "We've been married for thirty-one years, you know. If we wanted to do something different sexually, I don't think either of us would know where to begin."

It's a legitimate question, but one that also contains its own answer. Where you make love can make a difference. Try the living room instead of the bedroom, for example, a departure from the usual, and a starting point for your own imagination.

Most of us have sexual fantasies, although we don't like to admit it. The new permissiveness, for the most part, affects the young adult; the mature man or woman may feel that even thinking about a partner other than one's mate is a kind of infidelity. Psychiatrists and psychologists believe that sexual fantasizing is normal and healthy. Why not discuss fantasies with your mate, and act out those that appeal to both of you? Not every couple can do this, nor would every couple feel comfortable even discussing the idea. But many, to their surprise, find they can—if they make the effort.

Knowing what works for you sexually and what doesn't is important. Part of the reason that many people in their middle years today feel sexually dissatisfied is that our society has placed such a great emphasis on sex. Book after book and expert after expert, some legitimate and some self-styled, have appeared in the public spotlight to tell us how to live our sex lives.

Many people feel cheated. They grew up in a more rigid atmosphere, and now that the world is opening up sexually, they feel they have missed something. Once again, I recommend focusing not on what might have been, but on what can be. If erotic books and sexually explicit motion pictures stimulate you sexually, there is certainly ample opportunity to enjoy them.

There are others who don't like these things and feel that our society is too sexually oriented. Their opinion is equally legitimate. For all the expert (and nonexpert) advice on sex, we need to be reminded that sex is a very personal thing. What goes on between a man and a woman in intimate moments must be suited to that man and woman's tastes and desire. We can no more attempt to live out somebody else's expectations of what our sex lives should be like than we can attempt to follow some third party's taste in music or art. Sex is the most personal form of communication. Books and magazine articles can suggest, recommend, and broaden your horizons, but only you can determine what you like and what you don't like sexually.

Sex must be put in the proper perspective in a marriage. For some people, sex and love are synonymous. But tenderness, devotion, caring, and love are important, and essential to a good marriage. It is possible for some couples to have happy lives together without sex at all. If this pleases both partners, it is their business and their decision to make.

It has been my experience that the "ideal" relationship is rare indeed. Very few couples complement each other in all aspects—each partner enjoying all of the other's interests. But in over twenty years of practice, I have seen a lot of satisfied couples, and the secret common to them all has been compromise and contribution.

The medical community and the new breed of "sexologists" have done little research into the sexual habits of couples in their middle years and older, possibly out of the middle aged researchers' own embarrassment. Of the many "sex therapists" who have hung out an uneducated shingle in the past few years, few have much competence at all—much less the delicacy to deal with the complexities of climacteric sex.

Certainly there is no medical recipe for what guarantees a normal, happy sexual life at any given age. Knowing yourself sexually is important, and leads to satisfaction. But in discussing the "facts of life," we must face the truth that certain situations occur where other answers are needed. As a physician, I usually encounter sexual crises when the patient or couple involved has thoroughly exhausted every possible solution they can think of. I must approach each case with sensitivity, knowing that I am treating not only the sexual problem, but a patient or patients who are experiencing a mixture of anxiety, frustration, and desperation. For this reason, I recommend strongly that help be sought with sexual problems as early as possible. No matter how bad a problem seems, some answer can usually be found. But it is always easier to find a solution when you are calm—particularly in the area of sex, where pressure compounds any difficulty.

I greatly empathize with a patient of mine who had been through a most difficult year. She'd gone through the menopause, and then her husband's sudden death sent her into a reactive depression that I treated. A year later, Marion faced a different problem.

She'd worked through her grief, and the question she faced was what to do about her future.

"I have to admit that I feel uncomfortable discussing this with you," she told me, "but I really don't know where else to turn."

I assured her that she should feel relaxed, and asked what the problem was.

"It's sex," she announced. "I've come through the menopause, and I've gotten used to being without my husband, at least as used to it as you can get when you love somebody and lose him. I want to start living again, Dr. Parrish. I've begun thinking about sex."

I reassured her that it was normal and healthy, and she'd accepted her husband's death and mourned for him, and that sex was, as she'd put it, part of living again.

"Oh, I'm not ashamed or embarrassed," Marion told me. "I just don't know where to find sex."

I found that hard to believe. Marion was a very attractive woman. She had friends—couldn't they introduce her to eligible men?

"I don't want to meet eligible men," she explained. "At least not eligible for marriage. I wish my friends would stop trying."

Marion told me that her friends, all of whom lived in the same suburban community where she had a house, were already beginning to match her up with prospective husbands at dinners and parties. But she didn't want to marry, at least not in the foreseeable future.

"I want a sexual partner," she said, "but our little group is so closely knit that everyone knows everybody else's business. Several of my friends live on my street—I couldn't think of having an affair without their finding out. So I have the choice of marrying, which I don't want to do, or being a chaste widow for the rest of my life."

It was a problem, I agreed, but I was also able to come up with a suggestion. Why didn't Marion go to a club of some sort—cards, investments, or whatever suited her interests?

"I'm not a joiner," she answered, shaking her head.

I pointed out that she'd probably find other people who weren't joiners either, but who were in fact there to meet people, just as she was. There were even respectable "single again" groups holding regular social meetings. Among the widowers and divorced men who attended, I was sure she'd find someone she liked—and who wasn't pressured by mutual friends to propose marriage.

Still another solution for the widow or widower who finds socializing with friends of the late spouse too painful to be productive in terms of a relationship of any kind, is a change of scene. Discovering new places means discovering new people. Several years ago a very close friend of mine died in a car accident. We'd often gone to a restaurant that we both liked, and after her death I found I couldn't go through the door without feeling sad. One evening I went out with a group of people, and we went to that restaurant. I was determined to overcome my reaction, but it wasn't possible. Now, I've learned to avoid this particular place. It's something that I shared with somebody else I loved, and that is something I accept.

In reestablishing a sex life after the loss of a spouse, it's important that channels of communication be left open. No two people make love the same way, and expecting an exact "stand-in" for somebody you've lost is self-defeating. After years of sex with the same person, it's hard to start all over with somebody else. Remember that sexual communication, like any form of communication, must be worked at.

Illness or accident can also create sexual problems. Bill, the husband of a patient who fell and broke her hip, came to me shortly after the accident for advice.

"I feel like the biggest heel in the world," he said. "And I kick myself for it."

"For what?" I asked.

After a pause, he blurted it out. "Well, I'm a highly sexed man. Phyllis isn't to blame for her accident—I know that. First she was in the hospital and now she's home, but it's going to be a long time before we can go to bed together."

Bill was right. Phyllis had suffered a bad break, and it would be months before she could enjoy intercourse. I knew, too, that as a woman who had a successful management career, Phyllis wasn't the ideal invalid during her recuperation. Accustomed to being active and in full control, she was angry with herself and demanding of others.

"Sometimes I think of going to a prostitute," Bill told me, " and then I hate myself. I think of my wife, and all the pain and discomfort she has. But I think that maybe I could help her better if sexual tension wasn't such a problem for me."

Bill was being very honest—and very human. Deprived of sex, obviously an important aspect of the marriage, he was angry, in a sense, with his wife for not being able to provide it, and angry at himself for wanting it. I thought it over.

Perhaps extramarital sex would relieve the immediate problem, but Bill loved his wife. Guilt might complicate matters. And if Bill was a highly sexed man who had found fulfillment in his marriage, then Phyllis no doubt missed sex as much as he did. I asked Bill about her feelings, and he looked at me in surprise.

"You know, I didn't even ask her, Doctor. I thought that with her hip, it would be the last thing on her mind."

I advised Bill to bring up the subject, and to try using masturbation and fondling. He agreed—and that was the last I heard until several months later when Phyllis, back on her feet and back at her job, came in on her lunch hour.

"I wanted to thank you for your help," she began.

"You did your share," I reminded her. "I know it wasn't easy for a woman as active as you to be a patient."

Phyllis smiled. "It certainly was a lot easier after Bill had that talk with you. You don't know what it felt like, being in bed and in pain. I wasn't a woman anymore—I was a sick thing! Once Bill and I started having sexual relations, even though it was different, I felt so much better. I was able to let myself get well. And now, even though I'm fully recovered, our sex life has more variety."

During the middle years, illnesses and health problems can and do occur. There is nothing wrong in thinking about one's own sex drive, but it is important to remember that a husband or wife, though ill, may have similar feelings, coupled with a sense of guilt at depriving the other partner.

The problems of sex during the climacteric can be difficult, but they can be solved if efforts at understanding, communication, and honesty—both self and mutual honesty—are made. New advances in medicine help people to live longer and live healthier—and rather than an ending, the middle years can be the starting point of many more years of happy, sexually active life.

The Mind and the Middle Years

Psychic Instability and Psychotropic Treatment

———

Psychic instability is frequently the first sign of the climacteric. It is not surprising that emotional problems are so common at this time, for beginning in the middle years the mind—both the brain and the psyche—is attacked by a variety of forces.

Some of these forces are internal (changes in chemical, biological, and physiological makeup) and some are external (changes in life-style, family relationships, marital and working status, etc.). Assaulted from within and from without by new and different demands to face change and reorganize priorities, it is no wonder the mind becomes emotionally disordered. In the course of this chapter, we shall be discussing the difference between internal and external psychological disorders and the various treatments available to alleviate them. But first, let us take a look at some of the more common symptoms of these disorders as they manifest themselves in the climacteric.

Inflammable emotions, a peevish disposition, and

erratic moods are not uncommon during the many adjustments of middle age. These wide and unpredictable swings in moods in turn create tension in interpersonal relationships. Tension is further reinforced by free-floating anxiety and insecurity. All these symptoms shorten attention span and interfere with usual powers of reason and concentration.

Headaches, which have served many a woman (and man as well) as an acceptable excuse for emotional indisposition, are more frequent around the time of the climacteric. In women, these headaches have historically been associated with the menopause, and were thought to be of the "migraine," or vascular type. Now it is generally believed they are "tension" headaches. However they are classified, they are unwanted interferences.

Insomnia in the climacteric has its primary source in the disrupted rhythm of rest and wakefulness. Futhermore, flushes and sweats can interfere with sleep, as can anxiety and depression. Worry keeps the anxious man or woman tossing and turning for hours, while a depressed person, after only a few hours of rest, suddenly wakes to fitfully await dawn. Whatever its cause, insomnia disrupts normal emotions and performance. Aggravating, and aggravated by other symptoms, inadequate rest seriously complicates the climacteric. Sometimes it is so important that the physician must relieve it before he can treat the other symptoms of his patient.

Denied the restorative powers of sleep, a patient becomes even more aware of his low energy level and easy fatigability. The most common complaint in my office is: "I'm too tired to do half the things I should."

Biochemical and hormonal imbalance alone can reduce physical stamina. Couple these factors with the stress produced by physical symptoms, and it is clear how one's functioning in every aspect of life can be impaired during the middle years. Faced with the many problems that require decision and action, the climacteric patient may be incapable of dealing with them. Occasionally feelings of inadequacy and frustration make him overreact, becoming wildly aggressive or antisocial or simply behaving in a manner foreign to his own personality. Frequently, feelings of uselessness bully him into silence. Unable to find the reassurance he needs, he withdraws. He protects himself by limiting his exposure to threatening situations. This isolation offers additional "protection" against his anger toward others. As much as he needs to purge himself of this hostility, he is afraid his friends will withdraw what little sympathy they've offered. He becomes depressed.

Depression is one of the most common characteristics of the climacteric. What's more, it can become cumulative. The hormonal imbalances, physical symptoms, situational and personal problems can progress with time into the severe psychotic depression we term "involutional melancholia."

There are those in the medical profession who would deny psychological symptoms are related to the climacteric. On the other extreme, some doctors treat all the symptoms of the climacteric as psychosomatic, resulting solely from the patient's disturbed mental attitude.

For my own part, I'm a firm believer in the interaction of the mind and body. My three years of residency in psychiatry confirmed my impression that psychological disorders are by no means simply the result of unsolved complexes and unconscious conflicts. Without a doubt there are genetic and biochemical factors just as influential, perhaps more so. A psychological disorder most often results from a combination of factors: a genetic weakness predisposes an abnormal reaction to environmental stress, or a temporary biochemical imbalance in the brain can become "chronic" if the disturbing emotional stimulus is not removed or resolved.

In middle age such psychological disorders often become apparent for the first time. This is not to imply that the climacteric *must* have its psychological upsets. But the middle years are years of transition, and transition is rarely accomplished smoothly. We have already seen what happens to the body as it enters the fourth and fifth decades. And we have gotten some idea of how these changes in turn affect the mind. With the climacteric comes the sobering reality that it is later than we think.

The essence of the climacteric is a coming to terms with the new you. Though in the final analysis the climacteric is an individual phenomenon, there are several common themes. One predominating theme centers around the effect of the change in physical appearance; another around the limitations imposed by alterations in physiology; a third around the new role circumstances have created; and still another around reactions to the attitudes of one's friends and family. For these as well as others there is the common denominator of the mind, which is not only responsible for the various emotional reactions but also for integrating, resolving, and implementing the necessary steps to establish a new equanimity.

Though the mind is amazingly adaptable and has a formidable battery of defense mechanisms, periods of discord surface from time to time. Such a period of discord is often reflected in the signs and symptoms of the climacteric.

Brain chemistry is now recognized as being as important as external circumstance in creating state of mind. Brain chemistry may be even more important because when it is disordered it is more difficult to correct disrupting circumstances. Disordered brain chemistry impairs our ability to think and feel and therefore our ability to function. The brain cells, like any other cells, are dependent on a healthy metabolism. I believe that within the next decade it will be shown that most mental disorders are the result of abnormalities in this metabolism.

But barring inherent biochemical abnormalities of the brain or external factors that alter emotions and in turn brain metabolism, our state of mind is also affected by other changes in our body chemistry. Some changes are the natural result of the daily or seasonable ebb and flow of body functions. Some such changes undoubtedly contribute to the symptoms of the climacteric. Unfortunately, the chemical changes are difficult to translate into specific emotional conditions. I will try to describe these chemical phenomena in general terms, however, to give you some idea of the way they may affect your own mood or state of mind.

The most important chemical mediators are hormones. Their relative presence or absence is dependent upon the interaction between the nervous and endocrine systems which control their secretion. The master endocrine gland, the pituitary, for all practical purposes is a part of the brain and is directly and indirectly connected with areas and structures that affect most of our primary functions. Factors we have yet to understand, innate natural phenomena, act through the pituitary and nervous systems to both stimulate and inhibit the hormonal activity of the various endocrine glands. This close association between nervous and glandular systems has come to be known as the neuroendocrine system.

In terms of mental health, the hormones of the adrenal glands are probably the most important. They affect virtually every function of the body, and most importantly they buffer us against the effects of stress. We are all familiar with epinephrine, commonly known as adrenalin. In response to threatening situations, the adrenal gland accelerates its secretion into the blood and prepares us for flight or fight. The heart and respiratory rates increase, the blood pressure rises, and the metabolism is increased to furnish energy. The brain is stimulated, and we become excited and alert. Our actions are influenced more by our emotions than our reason.

Whether we interpret the stimulus wisely or foolishly, our response is based on instinct and experience. Should our neuroendocrine system fail to furnish us with the necessary adrenalin, we wilt or faint, or, in more critical situations, go into shock.

In response to stress the adrenals also increase their secretion of corticosteroids, the most familiar of which is cortisone. Their effects are not as dramatic as those of adrenalin, but they are just as important. Besides affecting such essential functions as carbohydrate, fat, protein metabolism and salt and water balance, they reinforce the functions of the cardiovascular system, the kidneys, voluntary muscles, and the nervous system.

A deficiency of the corticosteroids results in depression, irritability and irrational behavior. An excess can cause hyperactivity, euphoria, anxiety, and insomnia. Obviously, mental stability can be directly influenced by the neuroendocrine system.

The adrenals are not the only glands to react to stress. The male sex glands also affect responses in certain situations, as has been demonstrated by experiments with monkeys. For example, the amount of testosterone manufactured by a male monkey is greatly reduced when he is transferred from a familiar environment, in which his masculinity is clearly established, to one in which he is a stranger. His neuroendocrine system temporarily deprives him of this chemical force of masculinity, thus rendering him nonaggressive and less liable to attack by male members of the new group. (Happily his testosterone level bounces back when he is returned to his harem.)

A similar situation seems to affect men during the climacteric, when waning gonadal function often becomes a problem. How and why is still being explored. Though decreased testosterone secretion may protect a monkey in an alien environment, keeping him from being aggressive and offensive, the loss of the positive metabolic effects of testosterone can be detrimental in the middle-aged man. Not only does a deficiency weaken a man's physical and sexual prowess, it impairs his psychological attitude.

The psychochemical effect of estrogens is another exciting field of exploration. That it is intimately involved in the neuroendocrine system is demonstrated by the amenorrhea that results in times of stress, such as war and suspected, unwanted pregnancy. And there is hardly a woman who can deny the "moodiness" of the menstrual cycle. When the estrogen level is high, at midcycle, so is the mood, in marked contrast to the emotional indisposition of premenstrual and menstrual days when the estrogen level is low. Furthermore, as a general rule, women report that they have never felt better—on top of the world no matter what the circumstances in other parameters of their life—then when they were pregnant and estrogen levels were soaring. And physical symptoms aside, women started on ERT frequently report a remarkable transition from emotional discontent to a sense of well-being.

Aside from hormones, there are other chemicals that affect the brain. A few of the more important are sodium, potassium, sugar, and oxygen. Though these chemicals may have influenced our moods through our younger years, their importance is greater as we move into the middle years. With aging comes changes in our biochemistry that alter our mental attitude. As a result the chemistry of the brain no longer offers the support we have come to expect. Furthermore, those inexplicable changes in mood—the daily, monthly, and seasonal variations that are part of the body cycles—lose their synchrony. They become more exaggerated, and the lows seem deeper and longer. The effects of the various chemicals on mood cannot be discussed fully here, but a brief rundown will give the general idea.

Sodium affects the hydration of cells; too much can cause them to swell; too little, to shrink. Too much sodium could possibly account for some of the irritability of premenstrual tension, and too little for the anguish of a hangover. Excess of potassium is a possible explanation for the increased excitability of nervous tissue. Accumulation of this electrolyte results in an "overheating" of nerves, the blowing of mental fuses.

Sugar has long been associated socially, if not chemically, with mood. And now there seems to be scientific support for the terms "sweet disposition," "acid tongue," and "sourpuss." Excess sugar in the blood, diabetes, can cause a person to be irritable, nervous, and depressed. Too little sugar, hypoglycemia, can result in difficulty in concentration, wide mood swings, and acute anxiety attacks. The symptoms of these conditions can be so similar to mental disorders that the service of a psychiatrist, rather than an internist or endocrinologist, is often sought. But in these cases psychotherapy is not needed. Regulating their blood sugar restores their mental stability.

The subject of sugar introduces the subject of nutrition

and its relation to the brain and mental state. Obviously an undernourished brain does not function properly. There is evidence that certain nutrients, namely the vitamins, may, in large doses, exert a pharmacologic effect on the brain. The continued popularity of B-12 injections would seem to offer at least circumstantial support for this. And though the mechanism of action has yet to be explained, impressive results with megadoses of niacin and B vitamins have been obtained in some cases of schizophrenia.

The effect of oxygen on the brain, though not as chemical as the other factors we have discussed, is familiar to us all. An increased supply can produce a "high." Hyperventilation can make you giddy and faint; but controlled deep breathing, as in transcendental meditation, can be restorative. Oxygen deficiency, on the other hand, reduces cerebral functioning.

Organic brain disease due to arteriosclerosis is an unfortunate complication of aging. It is probably the primary cause of emotional irritability and aberrant responses to mental drugs in old people. Impaired circulation is most commonly recognized in memory disorders. Everyone reading this book knows a relative or friend who has a pitiful inability to recall recent events, but still an acute memory of the past. He cannot tell you what he had for breakfast, but he can tell you exactly what he was doing when the radio broadcast the end of World War II.

Our awareness and fear of this problem of "senility" can frequently be recognized in the jokes of middle-agers about their absentmindedness. Jokes they may be, but the concern itself can complicate the climacteric. Admittedly, halfway through life our memory seems to fail us more often. Words and dates do not come to the tip of our tongue as quickly as we want. We find ourselves in the middle of a room wondering what we have come to get. And repeated efforts to etch in our minds some new bit of knowledge end in frustration. Such experiences tend to make us doubt our mental competence. But only in rare cases is our brain or arteriosclerosis at fault. If we need to place blame, it must be placed on our psyche.

There is nothing to be ashamed of; the problem is simply a matter of the mind's having become overloaded to the point that it no longer sponges up anything new for the sake of absorbing it. If the matter is important enough, it will be remembered. We are not senile; we are preoccupied.

Preoccupation in the climacteric is a fact of life. Until now the years have been busy tumbling one over the other with growth and development, experiment and experience, recuperation from failure, and expansion of success. The future was what counted. In the climacteric the future is no longer some distant reward—or problem. It is here, and it needs firm decisions and plans, though we resent having to make them. The inevitable changes of life and living can no longer be postponed. We and our world are changing.

Besides having to adjust to chemical changes in the body and brain, the psyche is put on trial. No matter how much we have anticipated the changes, no matter how much we have intellectualized our acceptance of the new demands that come with age, we are unprepared. In spite of token concessions, superficial adjustments, even specific plans made in youth, the psyche is not ready for the jolt that can come from a look in the mirror, an attack of arthritis, an unexpected rejection, a moment of sexual inadequacy, and the realization that your next birthday is your fiftieth.

Your attitude becomes negative; you focus on the missed opportunities of the past rather than the promises of the future. Events of the present seem to conspire against you just when you have lost the resources that have customarily served as your weapons in battle. Your children give you problems; a recession or an inflation undermines your economic security; your spouse takes a lover; your job comes in jeopardy or your business fails in its potential. Suddenly everyone starts treating you in a manner "appropriate to your age." Your purpose in life seems to have lost its meaning and nothing new has come along to replace it. You may have considered the possibility that your circumstances would not always continue the same, but you never seriously believed they would conflict with your plans.

Yet here they are—circumstances that refuse to be ignored. These sources of stress may be as trivial as the expiration of your refrigerator, as important as the demands of a new job, as grievous as the loss of your mother, as unexpected as the death of your dog, as bleak as empty rooms, as distracting as debts, as minor as varicose veins, as serious as suspected cancer. Even good things, as welcome as they might be, can be troublesome because their demand for decision creates stress. To move or not to move; to accept or reject a promotion; to start to work or do nothing; to go on an expensive vacation or to stay home and recoup; to buy the fancy car you have always wanted or save for retirement.

Reversals, stresses, decisions, and adjustments all produce conflicts and these conflicts are the core of the emotional symptoms of the climacteric. Considering all that a middle-ager has to contend with in reorienting his life, it is amazing the climacteric is not usually more severe.

One of the most distressing symptoms of the climacteric is depression. Most of us suffer from some form of depression from time to time, but during the climacteric it is particularly hard to ignore. At this time of life, even if circumstances are favorable, it is difficult to avoid melancholy moods about what might have been and what can never be. There is a tendency to ignore the experiences of the past, the good as well as the bad, and to grieve for the things not done.

Not only the psyche but also the brain directs the mind into the haunts of depression at this stage of life. It has recently been discovered that beginning generally in the late forties there is a gradual reduction of a psychochemical factor that normally exerts an antidepressant effect on the brain cells. There is no known explanation for this phenomenon, so at present it must be considered another degenerative condition of aging. It could be considered the most important one, because the others can be tolerated as long as the spirits are high.

Because of the many factors that can cause depression—physical, psychological, chemical—it is often difficult to diagnose, and to treat. The interaction among these factors causes confusion, for both the patient and the doctor. It makes distinction between what is real and what is imagined difficult. Examinations and tests are usually more valuable for excluding a possible etiology than for finding one. A careful history and deductions from it along with the intuitive impression of the patient and the knowledgeable experience of the physician are sometimes invaluable in defining and managing a case of depression. This was true in the case of Peggy Graham, whose symptoms centered around a rather deceptive menopause.

An extremely intelligent and aware person, Peggy was almost completely thrown by the symptoms of her climacteric. In addition, she had a number of personal problems. Her mother had recently died and she was increasingly worried about the state of her father's health. Her husband's recent promotion to president of his company was demanding more and more of his time, and she was beginning to feel neglected. Their sex life was no longer satisfactory.

Peggy had come to me for a flu shot, but I could see there was something else troubling her. As is so often the case with a climacteric depression, her real problem was so confusing she hardly knew where to begin.

As she sat in my office I encouraged her to describe her symptoms—no matter how insignificant they might seem. Hesitantly, she began to recite a list that included fatigue, insomnia, apprehension, headaches, tension, "blue" moods, bouts of crying, palpitations, hot flushes, and irregular menstrual cycles.

I asked her if she was on the pill, or if she was taking estrogen in any form. She replied that her previous doctor had taken her off the pill about a year ago, when the first symptoms of her menopause appeared. "Come to think of it," she reflected, "most of my problems seem to have started then, although he gave me a thorough physical and told me I was in perfect health."

I asked if he had prescribed estrogen, and she said no. A picture of hormonal imbalance was beginning to shape up. As we have seen, an estrogen deficiency can create havoc in the body, not just physically but mentally. Estrogen is an important psychochemical, and a severe deprivation can result in psychic instability and depression.

Peggy's Estrogen Index confirmed my suspicions that she was suffering from such a deprivation. I prescribed ERT on a twenty-eight day cycle, just as she had had with the pill. I felt that this would correct the chemical imbalance of her neuroendocrine system and thus alleviate many of the symptoms of her depression.

A month later my decision was justified. All was in order on her complete examination. Her estrogen level was almost back to normal, and she was much more herself again. She was less fatigued, had had no more palpitations, had fewer flushes, and had not suffered a single crying bout. She was by no means completely over the hurdle, but the signs of progress were encouraging, and it would take more time for the ERT to take its full effect. She still had a few symptoms. Some were modified hangovers from months of hormonal imbalance, others were purely psychosomatic manifestations of the personal problems that still faced her. But she now seemed eager to control her problems rather than let them control her, and I felt sure she would more effectively cope with her psychosomatic symptoms once her psychochemical balance was completely restored to normal.

This is a good place to distinguish between "psychosomatic" and "hypochondriacal" symptoms. A hypochondriac looks for something to complain about, and the tone of his complaint seldom conveys the true nature of the symptom he describes. A psychosomatic symptom has a specific origin in an emotional problem. Transmitted by the nervous system, this emotional problem disturbs some organ or function.

One of the most distressing psychosomatic symptoms is fatigue. Today both in and out of my office the majority of people I encounter are tired. It is doubtful if extensive medical work-ups would find even in 25 percent a physical reason. A psychiatric evaluation would be more revealing, unearthing an etiology in probably half the cases. In a great many the diagnosis would be depression—however it might be described: boredom, melancholy, disillusionment, disappointment. When everything seems to go wrong, we lack the necessary motivation to set things right. Such a mental attitude, however, in our puritanical society is unacceptable. So we get tired.

Fatigue is particularly important in the climacteric.

Reasons to be depressed at this time of life are not difficult to come by. Peggy Graham's were valid, but they were aggravated both by the symptoms of her menopause and her hormonal imbalance. Once these were treated, her fatigue—and her depression—eventually disappeared. Unfortunately, not all cases of depression are as clear-cut and easy to treat as Peggy Graham's, as we shall see later in this chapter.

Another frequent psychological symptom of the climacteric is anxiety. It accompanies virtually every physical and mental disorder. There are a wide variety of types from free-floating to panic. It is manifested in ways as different as nailbiting and fear of riding escalators. Sometimes it is natural; sometimes it is imagined; either way it is often magnified. The slightest bit of anxiety is considered intolerable. Nursing it has become a way of life. Consider the billions spent on sedatives and tranquilizers. Witness the blooming popularity of transcendental meditation.

Some anxiety can be beneficial, a creative stimulus or a reason to take some positive action. Eliminating or submerging it has value only when it interferes with normal functioning, as in the case of Sidney Baxter, a patient of mine for many years.

Mr. Baxter was fifty-eight years old, ran a highly successful export-import business, which required his constant supervision, and had always had boundless energy. So I was surprised when he complained: "I can no longer complete a full day's work. I am not that old, but I can think of no other reason I should feel so washed-out. I'm questioning my physical and mental abilities from the time I open my eyes in the morning until I close them."

I was surprised at the way he looked. In the past I might have been concerned about his being too heavy around the middle and too flushed in the cheeks. Now I was concerned about his sallow complexion and drawn features. "Have you lost weight?" I ventured.

"Almost twenty pounds over the last six months, and not of my doing. Even when I have an appetite, once I start to eat it vanishes. I am so anxious that I jump when a door slams and I can't concentrate on the most important papers. The very thought of going into the office ties knots in the pit of my stomach."

It seems that Mr. Baxter was faced with the decision of expanding the business and enlarging the family fortune, or consolidating his holdings and reducing his own responsibilities. He was not cursed with ambition, but he had a normal amount. And with his wife's heart set on building a winter home in Jamaica, he could use the money. But he was tired of working so hard, especially when his efforts were unappreciated and unnoticed, especially by his oldest son, who showed no interest at all in the business. He wrote poems. The youngest son, still attending Harvard, did not seem interested in the business either.

I gave him a sympathetic ear and prescribed tranquilizers for his immediate symptoms, but his climacteric would not be resolved until he learned to cope with his anxiety. A crucial factor in the treatment of that anxiety was the management of his insomnia. Until his brain and body had the benefit of the restorative powers of sleep, he could neither feel nor think as he should.

A lot is said about sleep, but very little is known about it. Experience, however, has taught me several things I am certain cannot be refuted. "X" number of hours of sleep is needed to function properly. There is a maximum and a minimum daily or weekly requirement, which varies with each individual. Lucky is the one whose activities are not impaired with only five hours of sleep at night; he has the equivalent each week of one day more than the average person to live, learn, and love. Insomnia is a deficiency of an individual's minimum sleep requirement.

Unless Mr. Baxter anesthetized himself with alcohol, he averaged only three to four hours a night. After several weeks of this it is amazing he could function at all. His mind was not clear, numbed by the lack of sleep.

I believe that insomnia is a phenomenon resulting from a kind of overloading of the brain circuits during wakefulness. But what causes this overloading? Does some event of the day that refuses to dissipate continue to stimulate the brain cells? Possibly, and come the night it is too late to prevent this. Is it worry or caffeine?

Mr. Baxter had stopped drinking coffee, but there had been no noticeable benefit. However, the sleeping medicine I gave him was effective. Using it for a week revitalized his mental faculties. After that he used it only when necessary. But he recognized the value of sleep and the futility of trying to function and make important decisions without an adequate supply.

As a manifestation of unrest, anxiety can be physical or chemical, as in the case of shock or too much adrenalin. But most likely circumstances upset the psyche, which in turn upset the brain and the body. Hopefully the future will offer a simple explanation of anxiety. Ideally one simple chemical change will someday minimize the unpleasant aspects of anxiety and not otherwise disorder the mind or body. The drugs we use today to treat anxiety are in most cases effective. Unfortunately, their psychochemical effect is not specific enough. Side effects, both physical and mental, are frequent. But it would be impossible to imagine medicine and our society without psychotropic drugs.

Psychotropic medications are chemicals that correct

dysfunctions or improve the performance of brain cells. Altering the chemistry of the brain is intended to improve mental and physical health. It is not supposed to erase reality, only put it in its proper focus. Medical intervention in the realm of the mind is considered by most of us, whether or not we are aware of it, as unnatural. Perhaps the only psychotropic chemical that enjoys social acceptance is alcohol.

Psychotropic drugs can be broadly classified into two basic types: antidepressants and calmatives. First let us discuss the calmatives, which are used primarily to treat anxiety and insomnia.

There are several types of calmatives: hypnotics, general sedatives, selective sedatives, and tranquilizers. Hypnotics and sedatives are similar pharmaceuticals, frequently the same ones used in different doses depending on the effect desired. Their effect on the central nervous system is a general suppression of both the cerebrum, or "new brain" and the cerebellum, or "old brain." The reduced activity and excitability of the new brain limits excessive emotional responses. Suppression of the old brain slows down innate or learned reflex responses. In other words, sedatives and hypnotics dull the senses. This pharmacologic activity is used therapeutically to relieve hypersensitivity and hyperactivity of the nervous system. In small doses the effect is sedative; in larger doses, hypnotic, putting the patient to sleep.

There can be no doubt about the efficacy of these psychotropics in certain cases. Their value, however, has always been limited by the fact that their effect on the brain was not selective. Even with the most careful adjustment of dosage, attempts to simply calm the patient are frequently complicated by impairment of basic reflex responses.

It was only a quarter of a century ago that science discovered new agents for the treatment of anxiety and insomnia. There has been an ever-increasing number of these new psychotropic agents, but in the final analysis their activity is quite similar. In general they can be divided into two basis types: the selective sedatives and the tranquilizers. The selective sedatives suppress the entire central nervous system, but while they reduce the excitability of the new brain they do not impair reflex activity, either automatic or learned. The patient is sedated, and with increased doses usually becomes drowsy, but he can still muster his resources in time of need. The tranquilizers are even more selective. They modify overactivity without severely interfering with basic body functions.

This explanation and classification is perhaps oversimplified, but it gives a broad view of the chemical agents available to treat and control anxiety. Considering the many causes and manifestations of anxiety and considering the differences in individual biochemistries, there is a use for all of them. The problem is selecting the one that will best relieve the disturbing effects of anxiety in any individual case without invading other parameters of nervous activity.

The barbiturates, and some of the other older sedative-hypnotics such as chloral hydrate, are most effective when treatment demands a general calming of the central nervous system; the selective sedatives are most valuable in modifying abnormal behavior; and tranquilizers are preferred to help a patient adjust to a disturbing situation. The use of any of these requires discretion. None is without possible negative reactions. Side effects on various functions of the nervous system can negate the value of the therapy. A constantly dry mouth, drowsiness, or pupils that refuse to focus may be too great a price to pay for the ability to relax or suppress a curse. But perhaps even more important than these physical side effects are the psychological dangers.

These dangers, however, have sometimes been exaggerated, as in the prevailing opinion that as a society we are overtranquilized. It is true we are swallowing billions of psychotropic drugs a year. But perhaps the use of these drugs that modern science has discovered is based on a real need that our modern society has created. The answer to this question lies in analyzing whether in an individual case the drug is taken to help one deal with reality or to avoid it altogether.

It is a natural tendency to try to survive as painlessly as possible. But constantly taking a pill to avoid unpleasant feelings is ultimately self-defeating. Using an antianxiety medication to temporarily aid and abet one's natural resources, on the other hand, is as sensible as taking aspirin for a headache. It should not be considered a weakness of character.

It is perhaps unrealistic to hope that the future, tomorrow or twenty-five years from now, will not be fraught with problems that generate anxiety. But medical science is making great strides, and it is not unrealistic to hope that research will develop new psychochemicals that will effect peace of mind without physical side effects or psychological dangers. I have been working with a psychotropic that I feel has some of these qualities—diphenylhydantoin. It is not a new drug and has been used in the treatment of epilepsy for over thirty years. The action that makes it effective for epilepsy—reducing the excitability that explodes into muscular contractions—also appears to reduce emotional tension.

If we think of the brain as a series of electrical circuits (not an altogether elementary comparison), then an ideal drug is one that prevents the blowing of an overstimulated circuit. Diphenylhydantoin—or DPH—seems in some cases to provide such a fuse. Recent studies indicate that a nerve's abnormal excitability and its effect on the body and mind are a chemical reaction. No doubt a variety of chemical reactions can cause the overheating of neural tissues. Those that result from the accumulation of excess potassium seem to be controlled by DPH. I have been neither surprised nor discouraged that it did not work in all patients. But many patients with symptoms as varied as explosive tempers and impaired concentration have responded. For them DPH seems to do nothing more than correct some chemical imbalance. And in doing only that, it has approached the ideal of an antianxiety medication with negligible side effects.

By relieving the symptoms of anxiety, DPH reduces pressures and improves functioning. But it does not create a false sense of well-being that could be substituted for reality. For some patients it is needed only temporarily to correct some aberrant brain chemistry. For others with a chemical defect that seems to be inherent, its use can be compared to the hormone replacement therapies we have discussed.

I should note that use of DPH is not yet generally accepted by the medical profession. One valid reason for this scientific resistance is the difficulty in standardizing specific symptoms that call for its prescription. Since there is not yet a laboratory finding, or written or oral examination to define its psychochemical need, its use has to be based on therapeutic trial.

One indication for which I have not hesitated to try it is insomnia. Since the chemistry of sleep is so complicated, I can offer no concrete explanation for those cases in which it has been effective. An obvious possibility is a placebo effect, and in some cases this has no doubt been the secret of its success. But in other cases, where its efficacy has been repeatedly demonstrated, I have concluded that it cools the brain circuits so that the mind rests instead of being aggravated into unwanted wakefulness by an endless train of thoughts and emotional stimuli. This approach to the treatment of insomnia is not new. It was introduced with the tranquilizers.

The efficacy of tranquilizers in insomnia lies in their permitting a person to go to sleep. They relieve the mind of enough of its burdens so that the brain can succumb to the natural phenomenon of rest and recuperation. Hypnotics and sedatives force the brain into a dormant state. Though sometimes this strong effect is needed to relieve a person from the overwhelming cares of his life, the sleep is not all that restorative. If the effect of the hypnotic is brief, lasting only long enough to induce sleep, its effect is more salutory. It does not block out for the whole night the various levels of sleep, such as the dream phase, which seems necessary for the psyche to put its house in order. The mind needs the experiences of sleep as well as those of wakefulness to function properly. Eliminating these with constant or too heavy medication can distort reality.

The primary value of calmatives is their monitored use in helping cope with the symptoms of emotional stress— allaying anxiety that is distracting or overwhelming, inducing sleep when insomnia becomes physically or mentally debilitating, soothing irritability when it interferes with normal interpersonal relationships, and regulating an erratic or hyperactive nervous system when it aggravates the body's homeostasis.

The second broad classification of psychotropics is antidepressants. They generally operate on the two big hemispheres of the "new brain," acting as psychic stimulants to fight depression. Their effect on the cerebellum, or old brain, which governs the primal functions of life, is variable. Ideally they affect the mind, not the body.

The many faces of depression can be divided into two basic types: the reactive and the internal. The reactive depressions are exaggerated psychological responses to some external circumstance—an illness, a loss, a regret. It revolves around some situation that has a definable problem and a possible, though not always practical, solution. The psyche more than the brain is involved, though some changes in brain biochemistry have been noted in such cases. These changes are similar to those to be described in the internal depression, but they are not as severe nor their effects as widespread.

The internal depressions are chemical disorders in the metabolism of a group of neurochemicals called the catecholamines. It is thought that these bioamines are essential for the transmission of nervous impulses, especially across the synapses or junctions of nerve cells. The catecholamines are found throughout the brain, but are concentrated most heavily in the brain's limbic system, which helps regulate the emotions and such basic functions as sex and hunger.

There are many catecholamines, but the ones that seem to be particularly involved in depression are dopamine, norepinephrine, and serotonin. These compounds are not only similar to the hormones secreted by the adrenal glands, they are also important neurotransmitters in the neuroendocrine system. The action of these catecholamines in regulating moods and endocrine gland function offers scientific support for the clinical observation that the mind and hormones are interrelated. The disorder of one can be reflected in the disorder of the other, as in the menopause.

Sound evidence supports the theory that the

catecholamines are involved in depression. Drugs like reserpine (used in the treatment of hypertension) that reduce the concentration of the amines in the brain can cause depression. Patients with primary internal depression seem to have a deficiency of the amines as determined by the reduced amount of its metabolities, or breakdown products, excreted in the urine. And drugs that increase the concentration or inhibit the metabolism of the amines have an antidepressant effect.

The discovery of drugs that increase the catecholamines in the brain has been one of the most important advances in psychopharmacology. The first group of these antidepressants or "psychic energizers," as they are sometimes called, to be used clinically were the monamine oxidase inhibitors. They inhibit the activity of the enzyme monamine oxidase, which destroys the brain amines. Unfortunately, their effect was not limited to the emotional centers, and effective as they were in counteracting depression, their use has been limited by serious side effects. Fortunately, pharmacology has discovered another group of antidepressants—the tricyclics. By keeping the amines from entering the cells, the tricyclics increase their concentration at the synapses where they are needed.

The tricyclics are now the most common pharmaceutical therapy for internal depressions. They are not always as effective as patients and doctors would like. One of the reasons for this disappointment is the length of time, two to four weeks, for their full effect to be felt. Another is the side effects, in particular dryness of the mouth, visual disturbances, and drowsiness. These side effects usually pass and can be minimized by taking the medication in a single dose at night. And patience in waiting for them to correct the defect in brain chemistry is usually well worth the reward. There is an increasing feeling that these chemical compounds are more valuable in treating internal depressions than psychoanalysis.

The tricyclics have little benefit, however, in the treatment of reactive depressions. Circumstance, not chemistry, is at the root of these painful and increasingly frequent reactions to the vicissitudes of life. Time and an attentive ear seem the best therapy. There are, however, things that can be done to shorten the period of adjustment.

The most useful psychotropics in these cases are drugs that stimulate the brain. The best known of these are the amphetamines, chemical relatives of epinephrine, or adrenalin, and the catecholamines. But instead of correcting some chemical imbalance, the amphetamines produce a temporary state of euphoria. As welcome as it might seem, this false state of well-being is not infrequently followed by a depression as the medication wears off. Furthermore, the stimulating action on the central nervous system may cause undesirable effects, such as an increase in the blood pressure and palpitations.

But more than their side effects, their primary psychotropic effect, euphoria, has been responsible for their fall into disrepute. In analyzing the present negative attitude toward them, it is difficult to separate social factors from scientific fact. Our society has a basic fear of feeling good if it is not natural. And well it might, considering the daily tragedies resulting from the use of alcohol. Even taken proportionately, the number of people who have abused their lives taking amphetamines has been far less than those using alcohol.

No doubt it is better if we can cope with life on our own chemistry rather than with one that has been artificially created. But this is not always possible or practical. In selected cases psychostimulants are valuable therapeutic tools. In considering their use with a patient my basic consideration is their benefit in breaking the circular descent into the whirlpool of depression.

The most serious manifestation of a depressive reaction is withdrawal. Feeling rejected and angry at the world, a depressed person tends to lose interest in himself and life. The more he concentrates on his plight and his problems, the more depressed he becomes. And the more depressed he becomes, the less effort he makes toward adjusting to his situation.

These depressed people need involvement outside of themselves, something to distract them from their morbid thoughts or occupy their time. In such cases psychostimulants, given under medical supervision, can interrupt the crippling cycle of depression. The objective of the medication is not to produce a state of euphoria, but it frequently motivates the individual to help himself. If within a few weeks there is no indication of this desired response, the medication is discontinued. In cases where it is effective, it is tapered off as soon as there are indications that the patient can function on his own.

Depressions are a part of life. There is no way to avoid them. But there are ways to modify them, and such modification must be tailored to the individual case. No drug therapy is always completely safe and effective. But neither is the treatment of pneumonia. If there were ideal treatments for these conditions, there would be no need for the services of a physician. Admittedly, compared to antibiotics, psychotropics have in addition to the physical side effects, the possibility of habituation, a disorder I think the future will show to have deeper roots in abnormal biochemistry than in social maladjustment.

We are right to be concerned about the abuse of psychotropic agents, a concern that has now spread from the stimulants and sedatives to the tranquilizers. Though only a few people have the psychological or metabolic tendency to become dependent, the potential is always there. But the danger does not lie in restoring a previous state of calm or good humor; it lies in creating a false state of mind that unnaturally separates us from the reality of our lives. Doctors have been placed in the frequently uncomfortable role of deciding how good or bad a patient should feel. Frequently their personal opinions are reflected in their therapy.

Unfortunately, anxiety and depression rarely exist as isolated phenomena. They are usually mixed, though one is usually primary and the other a secondary, or complicating, phenomenon. This is important to recognize in outlining a regimen of psychopharmacologic treatment. Not infrequently, especially at the beginning of treatment, more than one psychotropic is needed—one for the primary condition and one for the complicating secondary ones. A calmative may have to be given along with an antidepressant and vice versa. This necessitates not only carefully titrating and balancing the drugs but selecting the combination that is most helpful for the patient and causes the least side effects.

In discussing the psychological aspects of the climacteric and their treatment, I have emphasized the chemical causes and psychopharmacologic treatment. In many cases I have learned this is the most direct approach. But I know its efficacy would be greatly reduced if I ignored the value of supportive counseling. In my sessions with these patients I try not only to give them the feeling that someone is interested, but that something can and will be done to help them. In addition I try to motivate them to experiment with different attitudes and become involved in activities that have not only a diverting interest but ones that will continue to be rewarding. Just because some old things are over and done with does not preclude finding new interests to give life meaning.

Spending time with patients suffering the trials and changes of middle life gives them an opportunity to express their true feelings without fear of reprimand. As they express their bitterness and disappointments, their improbable dreams and their regrets, I serve as a kind of converter that reflects these feelings back to them in a more acceptable form. In the process I sometimes unmask a previously undetected depression or I am able to point out a behavior pattern that has always worked against their having the kind of life they claim they long for. I also give the benefit of my knowledge, experience, and resources to help them resolve existing or prospective problems. It is amazing sometimes how what seems to be a simple solution to a problem has never dawned on the person who has been blinded by its seemingly endless complexities.

Most important, I try to introduce reality. The symptoms of the climacteric are frequently nothing more than the means of avoiding a coming to terms with one's life. It is almost as if suffering or complaining enough about it will make it go away. In such cases I sometimes calculatedly force them to deal with the cold, hard facts. Nurturing the past plants no seeds for the future. I point out that old age has advantages that youth conspicuously lacks. The most important of these is experience.

Hardly a person has not been able to point out some modus operandi that they have learned and refined that has served them well in the past. This, then, is a good way to start making plans for their new way of life. It might have to be modified to fit the new circumstances, but it is still a base from which to start. Some find new strength in religion; some develop a hobby into a business; some get involved in the lives of others; some simply learn to relax and enjoy the things they have never had time for.

In the final analysis coping with the climacteric is not just a matter for psychotropic drugs or psychotherapy, helpful as they might be. It is a matter of getting rid of the complications in your life so that you can concentrate on a new, realistic way to get the most out of coming years. Some dreams will have to be sacrificed and the mistakes of the past forgotten or turned to your advantage. One of the most important things you can do is to take advantage of every opportunity—even before the onset of the climacteric—to insure continued good physical and mental health.

The Best Is Yet to Be

The Benefits of Preventive Medicine

———

We've spent the bulk of this book identifying and explaining the climacteric as a medical problem—both physical and psychological—shared by all men and women. We've seen cases where the problem remains dormant as a result of good planning and fortunate circumstance or where a lack of symptoms conceals pernicious long-term degeneration. And we've discussed other cases where critical situations erupt, as immediately debilitating as a serious disease.

In this final chapter, our focus shifts. I want to discuss how every person can prepare for an inevitable phase of his or her life. How can you plan for *your* climacteric; how can you recognize its symptoms; how can you help treat it when it arrives?

But first let's look again at what the climacteric is all about. To begin with, it is not a disease, per se. Rather, it is a phase of life—a period of growth, if you will. A series of biological phenomena occur sometime between forty and sixty in all normal humans. These phenomena—

whether they are reflected in physical and emotional symptoms or not—define the climacteric.

Second, the biological changes of the climacteric can produce or contribute to a variety of disease processes. Chief among these for women is a deficiency disease, an insufficient—or even nonexistent—production of the vital hormone estrogen. Estrogen deficiency, in turn, has been shown to contribute to degenerative diseases ranging from osteoporosis to depression. The results of male hormone deficiency are less clearly defined, although it is certain that the biological changes in the male can produce a wide variety of alarming—even incapacitating symptoms.

And what of the psychological effects of the climacteric? For one thing, there are demonstrable neurochemical alterations that can occur during the climacteric, affecting the emotions. In addition, physical symptoms, coupled with the generational and social stresses common at this time of life, can seriously disrupt psychological well-being. In other words, if the biological changes do not in themselves produce emotional difficulties, they can leave an otherwise stable personality seriously vulnerable to external events. Trouble with, say, a difficult child can be coped with under normal circumstances; but occurring at a time when internal stress is present may produce an impasse.

So we see the climacteric is inevitable. What is not inevitable are its ill effects. These can be minimized— even eliminated.

But the decision is yours.

You can ignore change, but that is no insurance it will ignore you. You can hope for the best—and maybe you'll get it. Thousands of people pay no attention to the climacteric, or wouldn't know what the word meant if you asked them. Many will never suffer from their lack of attention. But many others will not begin to suffer until the damage is already done. It's Russian roulette played with stakes higher than simply life or death. For you won't die quickly from an improperly tended climacteric: you'll live on, plagued by an increasing array of conditions and diseases, many of which could be treated or might have been prevented. And *then* you'll die—probably earlier than you would have otherwise.

A pretty gloomy picture, isn't it? It needn't be: such a possibility should encourage you to use this book—not to mention your own good sense—to prevent the picture from becoming a reality in your own life.

Perhaps because of our enthrallment with youth and youthfulness, we've accepted the notion of adolescence as a difficult but natural period of physical and emotional change. It is preparation, the medical authorities tell us, for adulthood. We make allowances for emotional disturbances, we take the kids to the dermatologist for their acne—we *deal* with it.

So why then should we ignore this similar phase of life occurring some three decades later? The climacteric is also a period of adjustment and preparation. The two eras have much in common. We like to think of the education of our youth as a savings bank. The years of higher education are "deposits" on which the person may then draw for the rest of his professional life. The metaphor applies to the climacteric as well. We make our deposits in terms of medical attention and psychological adjustment during our middle years. The payoff comes after sixty-five or seventy, when our physical and mental health should be strong enough to allow us a vigorous and vital retirement.

Since the two periods are so similar, why should we pay zealous attention to the earlier, and little or none to the later? I think the answer is twofold:

First is our social attitude toward age. People are so fearful of old age that they try to avoid the necessity of preparing for it. And then middle age itself has taken on such a bad name that people almost *expect* it to be overwhelmingly awful. People have a vague sense of the serious disabilities that can occur during the middle years—and little or no real knowledge about what the disabilities are and how they can be treated. So many people resign themselves to ill health, whether they're fated for it or not. Those who do wind up with medical difficulties, feel almost vindicated. Those who escape are too relieved to question whether or not their fears were justified in the first place.

I'm not suggesting that people should assume their middle years will be a pathway of roses; overoptimism can sometimes be as nonproductive as pessimism. Instead, a general attitude of attention and care is called for.

The other reason we ignore the climacteric seems to me to be the fault of medical science. In the past century we've made phenomenal leaps in curing disease. But disease is not the only thing that can rob us of our health. And in our preoccupation with identifiable diseases for which there are specific, or sought-after, cures, perhaps we have neglected conditions that can have as serious effects—conditions like the climacteric.

Saving lives is not medicine's only concern: improving the quality of lives is equally important. We should be interested in preventing ill health as well as curing disease.

So perhaps as we talk about preparing for the climacteric, we would do well to begin by talking about you and your physician. The doctor-patient relationship is always an individual (and intricate) one, but one rule always applies: to get the best out of a doctor, one must first be a good patient.

Be informed about yourself in particular. The doctor is always going to know more about medical science than you do, but it helps if you attempt an understanding of your own body. Particularly as you approach the climacteric, it's important that you know what to look for. Laboratory testing can tell your doctor plenty about your health, but only you can tell him how you feel. Learn to be specific about your symptoms—where they're located, what they feel like, how long you've had them.

Be prepared for your examinations by keeping track of minor ailments you have in between visits to the doctor. If you've had a couple of colds, how far apart were they, how long did they last, where were they located? Any stiffness in the joints—and any obvious reasons, like overexertion, for them? General matters like your energy level, your sleep patterns, your sex life—all this is valuable data for your physician. If he doesn't inquire after them, bring them up. Remember that you and your doctor are in partnership for the care of your health, and both of you need all the help you can get. You live with yourself; he only sees you for a few hours.

The first rule of preventive medicine is to start early. Selecting a long-lived, physically strong and mentally sound mother and father is a good beginning. But not being able to do that we can still take advantage of our heredity and pay particular attention to avoiding the health problems that our ancestors and relatives suffered from. And do not wait until you are your parents' ages to start worrying about some condition that runs in the family. The younger you start, the better.

It has been suggested that the time to start preventive medicine is at birth. Starting good health habits as early as possible in life makes them natural and easier to maintain. Parents, however, should not assume that they have failed if children do not follow the suggested, sometimes enforced, regimens. But they should do everything they can to introduce and engender in their offspring everything they believe will make their future healthier.

The second rule is that it is never too late. No effort is ever wasted. The important thing is to make—and maintain—the effort.

And the third, and perhaps most important, rule is to be regular. Your preventive medicine program should include routine physical examinations. To make such routine examinations practical, I have established for myself some arbitrary rules, rules based on my own experience and conclusions from the experience of others. I do not hesitate to change them as circumstances indicate, and I try to adjust them to the changing times and techniques. But following a structured system make the examinations easier for me and my patients.

For patients under forty my examination includes first a history—his whole past if it is an initial examination or an interim history if it is a follow-up examination. Either way I do not rush because it is important to learn as much as I can and it is important that the patient express himself fully.

The physical examination is based primarily on what I can see, feel, and hear. Temperature, pulse, respiration, weight and height, and visual acuity are routine. So are rectal examinations, pelvics in women, evaluation of lung capacity and testing for increased ocular pressure. I think an annual X-ray of the chest is important, but I do not do electrocardiograms as frequently as that. Blood counts screen for anemias, infections, and abnormal cells; blood chemistries and a urinalysis screen for dysfunctions in the kidneys, liver, and thyroid and for abnormalities in sugar, fat and salt and water metabolism.

Examination of cells scraped from the cervix are also routine because cervical cancer can occur early in life. Fortunately, it is one of the easiest malignancies to treat, and early detection results in a 90 percent cure rate. Similar methods for collecting and examining cells to look for any that are alarmingly different in appearance (cytology) are being developed to look for other cancers. One of these that is now being refined is examination of the sputum for possible malignant cells. I encourage smokers of all ages to have this done.

At, or soon after, forty I recommend a more thorough examination. Additional tests are EKGs taken at rest as well as during and after exercise; upper GI series and barium enemas, sigmoidoscopy, mammography, and more extensive examinations of the urine and blood. Although it would be ideal, I do not routinely suggest all of these annually, but every three to four years. I do suggest interim examinations similar to that outlined for younger patients.

After fifty the tests outlined above would be ideal on a yearly basis. And these should be supplemented with other procedures that might be dictated by the patient's hereditary background, way of life, occupation, and physical complaints. I have already discussed in previous chapters some of the things that can be done to detect at an early date signs of degenerative changes. Any hint of one of these changes should be followed up immediately. That is the purpose of the preventive medical exam—to correct or modify any disease or degenerative condition before it has exacted its toll.

I will not say that the examinations as I have sketched them here are perfect for everyone. Each doctor has to make his own decisions. Here I might bring up the delicate matter of your satisfaction with your physician. If you are dissatisfied, you may want to consider changing.

But think first about the reasons for your dissatisfaction. Is the doctor at fault or are you? If you feel your doctor doesn't give you enough information, have you tried asking him? If you've had to wait for an appointment, try remembering if you've ever kept the doctor waiting— and been responsible for throwing off his other scheduled patients as well.

Maybe trouble with your physician is just a temporary matter. Perhaps you have a specific problem that you don't feel he's dealt with as well as you'd like. In such a case, other arrangements can be made. A woman seeing a general practitioner, for example, who is hesitant to start her on estrogen replacement therapy can always request another opinion. Her doctor can suggest a specialist—a gynecologist, say—who might understand her concern better. In any case, particularly where serious health matters are concerned, a second opinion is never a bad idea. If nothing else, the patient is reassured that the first doctor is indeed making the wisest decisions. And no modern physician should take any offense at such a request.

But if you just cannot generate any confidence or enthusiasm for your doctor, then I can only say leave. Everyone should have a physician in whom he has complete faith, particularly as one gets older. The best idea is to be able to turn over complete responsibility for monitoring your health to a single doctor. He should send you a date for regular examinations, keep complete records of your medical history, and be in charge of recommending other physicians or specialists when your need indicates.

Without a regular physician, you can too easily put off annual exams or ignore a problem that crops up, assuming, as is natural, it will "go away." When you feel bad, your doctor should know about it. No one likes a constant complainer, of course—that's not being a good patient at all—but your doctor will respect your interest in your health. And if a situation should arise where your doctor can find nothing wrong but your symptoms persist—go back. And go back again until your questions are answered, or get another opinion. It's more than a matter of "the squeaking wheel gets the grease": your doctor may be dependent on you to tell him exactly how serious your condition is. Do not cry wolf at every temporary indisposition you cannot understand. But remember it is your health and no one is going to attend to it as well as you.

What this all boils down to is nothing more than taking advantage of what medical science can offer you. Particularly now, as medical science shifts its concentration from the "cure," as I mentioned earlier, to prevention, relief from the ill effects of the climacteric is increasingly a reality. To deny yourself expert medical care during the middle years is to shortchange your own health—both now and in the future.

On the subject of medical care, I might also add that part of preparation for the climacteric era should include a review of your medical insurance. It's a fact of life that health problems occur more frequently during the middle years, and increasingly in later years. Don't add financial insecurity to the burdens of ill health.

The issue of top quality, ongoing medical supervision aside, what's a man or woman facing the climacteric to do? Sit around and wait for symptoms? Absolutely not—and that includes not measuring your own situation by your neighbor's. Never fall into the trap of monitoring your own health with secondhand information. Contrary to popular belief, men are as likely to pick up misinformation in this manner as women—and are just as likely to suffer the consequences. Just because the man next door describes his pains in the back exactly as you would your own does not allow you the liberty of appropriating his diagnosis.

This warning applies as well to the case histories in this book. Perhaps you recognize some of your own symptoms in the story of Mrs. De Marina or Dayton Killibrew. But your own case history is as unique as these. Only a physician can make a qualified diagnosis. Self-diagnosis, whether from a television drama or the morning paper, is a serious mistake. It could distort your own or even your doctor's objective observation—and in doing so delay identification of the real problem.

Instead, keep an open mind while on guard for the first symptoms of the climacteric. Look for any changes—physical or psychological—from your own personal norm. Keep a notebook, if you like, and record your observations. Include specific symptoms, time of occurrence (Do they usually occur in the morning or evening or after a big meal?), and their duration. When you feel that a specific change has indeed occurred, your record, whether mental or written, will be valuable to your doctor.

This attention may seem somewhat morbid, and I certainly don't suggest that you spend an undue amount of time watching yourself. You'll know when something of note is going on, so you needn't anticipate problems before they arise.

Your time would be much better spent on positive programs of physical betterment. For example, take that notebook and record every cigarette you smoke and every drink you take. Then—just for fun, as it were—figure a day of your life lost for each carton of cigarettes you smoke. Or think about what's happening to your liver every time you take more than two drinks in a single day. Then maybe add up the financial cost of your cigarette and/or alcohol habit. Consider how much money you could be stuffing under the mattress for that retirement home you've dreamed of.

Better still, modify or quit your poor health habits, right now. Not just alcohol and cigarettes, either. How about your cholesterol level? Your doctor can tell you from your laboratory reports how high your cholesterol and other blood lipid levels are. If indicated, see what you can do about cutting down on whole milk (the skimmed is quite tasty once you get used to it), eggs, and animal fats.

While looking at your diet, see what you can do about cutting down on your salt intake. If you have a husband who for years has unwittingly insulted your cooking by salting his food before even tasting it, now is the time to stay his hand—and for medical reasons, not out of pride. Too much salt—and almost all Americans are guilty of this—is a prime contributor to heart disease.

In general, try for sensibility in your diet. Dine lavishly, if you want, on lean meats and fresh vegetables, but reduce your intake of starches and fats. And don't forget roughage: constipation is a serious problem for many in the middle years and fruits and leafy vegetables are essential.

Even with the best diets, vitamin supplements are a good idea. Though its effects have yet to be proved, I do not discount the possible benefits of what is known as "megavitamin therapy." Taking essential food elements in amounts much greater than the known daily requirements may exert some positive biochemical effect. But I object to its becoming an obsession. One patient took eighty-three different pills a day. Besides being the cause of the indigestion about which he complained, the excess vitamin A, which the body stores in the fat, could be dangerous. I suggested he be more selective.

First and foremost in a supplemental dietary regimen is a strong vitamin-mineral combination to insure against any deficiency of a known essential element. Then for patients interested in trying to improve their biochemistry and possibly preventing some of the degenerative changes of time, I recommend large doses of vitamins B and C, which are water soluble and difficult for the body to store. I give particular emphasis to B-12 and niacin. I also include in my "antistress" regimen a calcium-magnesium combination and vitamin E. I can't "prove" the benefits accruing to my patients taking these vitamins in large doses—but I can testify to the lack of ill effects. Sound your physician out on vitamins. Scientifically he may be skeptical, but practically he will probably agree they will not do any harm and may offer some unexpected benefit. Just make sure they are fresh.

As you review your diet, which includes your calorie intake, take an equally hard look at your output. Regular exercise is as important during the climacteric as at any other time of life. Too many people think that age exempts them from all but essential physical activity. This is a dangerous misconception. Exercise not only improves the overall state of your health but increases your energy level in other areas. Then, at such time as climacteric symptoms develop, the sustained program of exercise you have undertaken will be an important factor in your ability to overcome their effects. Besides, the psychological benefits of being in good physical shape are immense. It's true that when we look better, we feel better—and not all of the sags and flabs of middle age are the result of gravity and time. Good muscle tone can do as much as cosmetic surgery to firm up your body.

How you get your exercise is unimportant, as long as you remember that overexertion can be as counter-productive as underexertion. Jogging has become a popular pastime, but if you're just starting out, your good sense will tell you not to begin with a five-mile jaunt.

Whatever form of exercise you choose, the important thing is to start out reasonably and *keep it up*. Sedentary ways can become a vicious circle: the less exercise you get, the less you're able to withstand. Be sensible, and be regular; fifteen minutes a day may be enough to start with—and better for you than three hours every other week.

Activities involving other people are a good idea (and I don't mean canasta!). Tennis, golf, dance class, and social sports provide not only a good opportunity for exercise, but serve the purpose of keeping you socially active. The temptation is strong during any troubled period of life to withdraw into ourselves, and it must be resisted. This is a matter of mental attitude.

Proper attitude is crucial for a problem-free climacteric. Physical care—with your doctor and on your own—is only half the battle. You should take reassurance from the steps you've taken and the plans you've made to keep yourself in good physical shape. But don't stop there: use the insight and experience you've gained in half a lifetime to take stock of where you've been and where you're going.

The middle years are a good time for a little applied selfishness—think of your own needs first, for a change. Chances are the obligations of parenthood are, if not completed, at least less a matter of day-to-day concern. Your professional situation, your home life, your social world, your patterns of daily life, your likes and dislikes—all these factors are becoming less likely to change. This thought might not be appealing, particularly if you are dissatisfied with some of these aspects of your life. So try to liven them up, improve them but do not risk any basic stability. Instead use these stabilities as a platform to know yourself better, and broaden your special interests.

It's hard to get a clear view of a landscape from a quickly moving train; but a stop at a station allows you to get out, stretch your legs, look about you. There is perhaps no better time or place than the climacteric to make the rest stop, even change trains, provided you know where you are going and how you are going to get there. Just remember you can't go back to where you started.

First, you're going to have to make some resolution with your own past. Failed goals, unrealized dreams, and all the things that never quite turned out as you expected—or hoped—now's the time to get some perspective on your personal history. It is not as hard as you may think to make a convincing case that everything that's happened to you, good or bad, has been ultimately for the best. This positive reconstruction of your past is a far more rewarding mental exercise than the endless circle of worry. Most important is the simple realization that mistakes of the past are valuable only insofar as we can learn from them.

Remember, that old saw about "if I knew then what I know now" works two ways. You *do* know now, so apply that knowledge to the only field where it can do any good: the present. And through the present, the future.

The future must always be approached with caution, and never more so than when we feel our future is not so open-ended as it once was. Let's face it: gambling is a privilege of youth.

Your decisions will be more thoughtful, and rightly so. You have more at stake as well as more experience to take into account.

But don't allow yourself to be paralyzed by decisions. The middle years are not the time to burrow inside yourself, to call a halt to life. By all rights, your mental powers should be at their sharpest. Your ability to make decisions is surer than ever before; changes—even major ones—are still a possibility, and your careful decisions should allow you to make the most of them.

Don't be paralyzed either by feelings that you're "too old." You may be too far along to be crowned Miss America and you may no longer qualify for competition on the "College Bowl." But you can still take up new hobbies, develop new interests and friends, even start a new career. (This last may be more difficult than it should be: businesses have shown an increasing unwillingness to hire mature personnel. But you can fight back—"equal opportunity" means just that—and if they don't know what good experience they're missing, you tell them!)

Perhaps you should take care not to involve yourself constantly in activities and associations that make you unhappily aware of your age. Friendship with younger people has its rewards—fresh attitudes, different opinions—but as a steady diet it can make you more jealous than stimulated. Just for balance, elect sometimes to be the junior member of a group yourself.

I don't mean to imply that your age is anything to be ashamed of. Far from it: the standard situation-comedy joke of the woman who refuses to tell her age is a sad commentary on contemporary attitudes. You have every right to be proud of your age. You've lived each of your years to the best of your ability—which, judging from the climbing suicide rate among youth, is more than many are capable of.

Your inner satisfaction should express itself in the way you act, even in the clothes you wear. "Appropriate" is the key word here. You should be delighted to "act your age," and to keep your activities, your dress, your makeup and hairdo appropriate to your years. To do otherwise—whether following the latest teenage makeup fad or socializing exclusively with members of a younger generation—is to fool only yourself.

"Appropriate" should not in any way limit your behavior or activity—you alone can decide what's appropriate for you. It is what is comfortable to you. The same qualification applies to any definition of "middle-aged" that restricts your personal freedom. There is no set standard of behavior for the middle years, only your own. Labels work well for canned goods in the supermarket, but have no place in individual life-styles. An objective look at your own life—your grooming, your associations, your activities—can tell you more than any self-designated authority about what's "right" for your age. If nothing else, you can rely on one of the few invariables of human society: your best friends *will* tell you.

And when they do, listen. Reject their advice, if you like, but show them the respect of listening. You may need all the support you can get, whether from friends or family, if you should suffer from a rough climacteric. If you do, you'll want your friends to listen to you.

Many physicians don't like the idea that their patients exchange experience and information; I can understand the concern. As I cautioned earlier, self-diagnosis, like a little knowledge, can be a dangerous thing. Still, I think it's important that patients feel comfortable about sharing their experience—particularly with a subject as ignored as the climacteric.

The climacteric, and the fears to which it gives rise, have been shut off from the public eye too long. Much of the ignorance is doubtless willful: since its most obvious symptom, the menopause, is both female and sexually related, our Victorian hangover has not seen the subject as fit for public consumption. Hopefully, such attitudes are evaporating, and our newfound taste for candor will find its way to an appropriate subject—the human body and how it works.

In addition, now that the climacteric is being recognized to affect men as well, the medical establishment (overwhelmingly male) is more likely to sit up and take notice!

Men may also find themselves with more than a twinge of jealousy over the advantage that estrogen replacement therapy offers to women. Estrogen is the closest thing to a "fountain of youth" that science has yet discovered. Not only does it relieve and prevent the common symptoms of the climacteric change, it forestalls much of the degeneration we associate with "old age." When combined with a rigorous program of medical attention and personal care, it can keep a woman vital long beyond the time allotted by Mother Nature.

Studies published within the past five years indicate even greater benefits. Aside from the prevention of osteoporosis and genital degeneration which we've discussed before, evidence supports the idea that estrogen therapy promotes a general sense of well-being. I'm confident that further research will unlock other, if not similar, therapies for men.

Already advances in the psychotropic drugs have provided relief from anxiety and depression for both men and women. Thirty years of success with a Romanian "revitalizing" drug trade-named Gerovital is now being tested, on a careful experimental basis, in this country. Consisting of a chemically altered form of procaine, commonly used as a local anesthetic, its exact mode of action is still being studied. And before the Food and Drug Administration releases it for use it wants proof that it does not harm and it has at least one reproducible benefit. Investigative research is collecting an impressive amount of proof that it beneficially affects the biochemistry of the brain. By inhibiting the destruction of the bioamines which prevent depression, it modifies our attitude and ability to cope with the aging process. If future research proves that it does this and nothing more, it will receive a prominent place in the medical armamentarium. Any other benefit, of which many have been reported, will be an added blessing. So for now we can all hope that it is the first of a continued development of treatments to make the later years as vital as the earlier ones.

But don't count on any future medical miracle to ease the stress of the climacteric. Instead, take advantage of the miracles science has already made available to you. These and the inner resources you can muster can be surprisingly effective. And don't forget, there is no better weapon to combat the trials of the climacteric than a sense of humor.

What happens with your future depends on how you handle yourself. And this is a matter of your overall attitude and the actions you take. It is a matter of evaluating and accepting reality. You must appraise your present resources, then as realistically as possible evaluate your future. Chances are the general course you take will fall under one of two main categories—security or growth.

Those who elect security feel they have gotten as much out of life as can reasonably be expected. Or perhaps their life so far has by no means been all they wished, but they feel they would jeopardize what they have in attempting to get more out of the future. So they begin to husband their resources. They avoid situations that might make them vulnerable to crises with which they can't cope or to injuries from which they couldn't recover. This doesn't mean they develop no new interest in life, but the ones they do take on are realistic and safe. Financially and emotionally, they use the years of the climacteric to secure a comfortable and happy future.

Those who elect growth feel that their life is unfulfilled and want to improve it. Or possibly their past has been so rewarding they simply want to continue to reap the benefits of new experiences. These people feel sufficiently secure in themselves that strange and hazardous situations do not intimidate them. They have no intention of giving up a cherished dream even if seeking it involves sacrifice and danger. They are constantly stimulated by the thousands of opportunities that life has to offer.

Whichever course you take, the first thing you must do is recognize where you are. And second, you must work at developing a positive attitude toward where you are going. If you can't cope alone, get help. The worst thing you can do is ignore or deny the inevitable changes that come with middle age. Your future is at stake. It's going to be different and you can make it interesting—ideally finding a happy medium of growth and security. Don't spend the next part of your life collecting "ifs." And most of all, don't let Father Time become your unsympathetic master.

The climacteric is a period of challenge and reevaluation. Do not be afraid to make the most of it. If you are willing to reap the rewards of your experiences, it can be a time of self-discovery and constructive growth. The trials of youth are behind you. Some of the best years of your life lie ahead.

Index

About the Author

A graduate of Louisiana State University School of Medicine, Dr. Parrish served his internship in New York City, followed by a year's residence in pathology at New York's Roosevelt Hospital. On the staff of New York Medical College, he worked in endocrinology with Dr. Max Goldzieher, a pioneer in the field, and concurrently served as a medical director at Ayerst Laboratories. After several years of private practice, Dr. Parrish completed a residency in psychiatry at Bellevue and Manhattan V.A. hospitals. For seven years he has been a consultant for the Dreyfus Medical Foundation on the use of diphenylhydantoin as an emotional stabilizer; his study now includes almost 1,000 patients. In New York, where he has a private practice in general medicine and psychiatry, Dr. Parrish continues to focus his unique qualifications on estrogen deficiency, preventive medicine, and the special problems of the climacteric.